Neuromuscular Disease Management and Rehabilitation, Part II: Specialty Care and Therapeutics

Editors

NANETTE C. JOYCE
CRAIG M. MCDONALD

PHYSICAL MEDICINE AND REHABILITATION CLINICS OF NORTH AMERICA

www.pmr.theclinics.com

Consulting Editor
GREGORY T. CARTER

November 2012 • Volume 23 • Number 4

ELSEVIER

1600 John F. Kennedy Boulevard • Suite 1800 • Philadelphia, Pennsylvania 19103

http://www.theclinics.com

PHYSICAL MEDICINE AND REHABILITATION CLINICS OF NORTH AMERICA Volume 23, Number 4
November 2012 ISSN 1047-9651, ISBN-13: 978-1-4557-5332-1

Editor: Jessica McCool

Reprints. For copies of 100 or more of articles in this publication, please contact the Commercial Reprints Department, Elsevier Inc., 360 Park Avenue South, New York, NY 10010-1710. Tel.: 212-633-3812; Fax: 212-462-1935; E-mail: reprints@elsevier.com.

Physical Medicine and Rehabilitation Clinics of North America (ISSN 1047-9651) is published quarterly by Elsevier Inc., 360 Park Avenue South, New York, NY 10010-1710. Months of issue are February, May, August, and November. Business and Editorial Offices: 1600 John F. Kennedy Blvd., Suite 1800, Philadelphia, PA 19103-2899. Customer Service Office: 3251 Riverport Lane, Maryland Heights, MO 63043. Periodicals postage paid at New York, NY and additional mailing offices. Subscription price per year is $263.00 (US individuals), $459.00 (US institutions), $140.00 (US students), $320.00 (Canadian individuals), $598.00 (Canadian institutions), $200.00 (Canadian students), $395.00 (foreign individuals), $598.00 (foreign institutions), and $200.00 (foreign students). Foreign air speed delivery is included in all *Clinics* subscription prices. All prices are subject to change without notice. **POSTMASTER:** Send address changes to *Physical Medicine and Rehabilitation Clinics of North America*, Customer Service Office: Elsevier Health Sciences Division, Subscription Customer Service, 3251 Riverport Lane, Maryland Heights, MO 63043. **Customer Service: 1-800-654-2452 (US). From outside of the United States, call 314-447-8871. Fax: 314-447-8029. E-mail: JournalsCustomer Service-usa@elsevier.com (for print support); JournalsOnlineSupport-usa@elsevier.com (for online support).**

Physical Medicine and Rehabilitation Clinics of North America is indexed in *Excerpta Medica, MEDLINE/ PubMed (Index Medicus), Cinahl, and Cumulative Index to Nursing and Allied Health Literature.*

Printed in the United States of America.

Contributors

CONSULTING EDITOR

GREGORY T. CARTER, MD, MS
Department of Clinical Neurosciences, Providence Medical Group; Hospice and Palliative Care Services, Providence Health Services, Olympia; MEDEX Division, University of Washington School of Medicine, Seattle, Washington; Department of Physical Medicine and Rehabilitation, University of California Davis, Sacramento, California

GUEST EDITORS

NANETTE C. JOYCE, DO, MAS
Assistant Professor, Department of Physical Medicine and Rehabilitation, Co-Director, ALS Clinic, Researcher, UC Davis Institute for Regenerative Cures, University of California Davis Health System, Sacramento, California

CRAIG M. McDONALD, MD
Professor and Chair, Department of Physical Medicine and Rehabilitation; Professor of Pediatrics, University of California Davis School of Medicine; Director, Adult and Child Neuromuscular Disease Clinics, Director, NIDRR Rehabilitation Research and Training Center in Neuromuscular Diseases, University of California Davis Medical Center; Director, Neuromuscular Disease and Spina Bifida Programs, Department of Orthopaedic Surgery and Rehabilitation, Shriners Hospital for Children, Northern California, Sacramento, California

AUTHORS

ALLISON L. ABRESCH, DO
Department of Family Medicine, Good Samaritan Hospital, Corvallis, Oregon

HUGH D. ALLEN, MD
Professor of Pediatrics and Medicine, The Ohio State University College of Medicine; Member, Center for Gene Therapy Research Institute and Staff Cardiologist, The Heart Center, Nationwide Children's Hospital, Columbus, Ohio; Presently, Professor of Pediatrics (Cardiology), Baylor College of Medicine, Texas Children's Hospital, Houston, Texas

JOSHUA O. BENDITT, MD
Professor of Medicine; Director of Respiratory Care Services; Director of Medical Intensive Care Unit, University of Washington Medical Center, Seattle, Washington

MARLIA M. BRAUN, PhD, RD, CSSD
Department of Food and Nutrition Services, University of California Davis, Sacramento, California

KATE BUSHBY, MD
Professor of Neuromuscular Genetics, Institute of Human Genetics, International Centre for Life, Central Parkway, Newcastle upon Tyne, United Kingdom

GREGORY T. CARTER, MD, MS
Department of Clinical Neurosciences, Providence Medical Group; Hospice and Palliative Care Services, Providence Health Services, Olympia; MEDEX Division, University of Washington School of Medicine, Seattle, Washington; Department of Physical Medicine and Rehabilitation, University of California Davis, Sacramento, California

PAULA R. CLEMENS, MD
Associate Professor, Department of Neurology, University of Pittsburgh; Neurology Service, Department of Veterans Affairs Medical Center, Pittsburgh, Pennsylvania

EDWARD M. CONNOR, MD
Professor of Pediatrics, George Washington University School of Medicine; Director, Office of Innovation Development; Professor, President and CEO, ReveraGen Biopharma, Rockville, Maryland

JESSE DAMSKER, PhD
ReveraGen Biopharma, Rockville, Maryland

JONATHAN FINDER, MD
Professor of Pediatrics, University of Pittsburgh School of Medicine, Division of Pulmonary Medicine, Allergy and Immunology, Children's Hospital of Pittsburgh of UPMC, Pittsburgh, Pennsylvania

KEVIN M. FLANIGAN, MD
Professor of Pediatrics and Neurology, The Ohio State University College of Medicine; Center for Gene Therapy, Research Institute, Nationwide Children's Hospital, Columbus, Ohio; Wellstone Muscular Dystrophy Cooperative Research Center, Rochester, New York

KEVIN J. GERTZ, PhD
Department of Rehabilitation Medicine, University of Washington School of Medicine, Seattle, Washington

MUNISH C. GUPTA, MD
Professor, Co-Director of Spine Center, Chief of Orthopaedic Spinal Disorders Service, Department of Orthopaedic Surgery, University of California Davis, Sacramento, California

LAUREN P. HACHE, MS, CGC
CINRG Operations Manager, Center for Genetic Medicine, Children's National Medical Center, Washington, DC

JAY J. HAN, MD
Co-Director of the MDA Clinic; Associate Professor, Department of Physical Medicine and Rehabilitation, University of California Davis, Sacramento, California

ERIC P. HOFFMAN, PhD
Professor and Chair, Department of Integrative Systems Biology, George Washington University School of Medicine; Director, Center for Genetic Medicine Research, Children's National Medical Center, Washington, DC; ReveraGen Biopharma, Rockville, Maryland

TIMOTHY M. HOFFMAN, MD
Associate Professor of Pediatrics, The Ohio State University College of Medicine; Staff Cardiologist and Director, Cardiac Transplantation, The Heart Center, Nationwide Children's Hospital, Columbus, Ohio

MARK P. JENSEN, PhD
Professor and Vice Chair for Research, Department of Rehabilitation Medicine, University of Washington School of Medicine, Seattle, Washington

NANETTE C. JOYCE, DO, MAS
Assistant Professor, Department of Physical Medicine and Rehabilitation, University of California Davis Health System, Sacramento, California

WENDY LIN, MD
Associate Physician, Department of Pediatrics, University of California San Diego, San Diego, California

SUKANTA MAITRA, MD
Department of Orthopaedic Surgery, University of California Davis Medical Center, Sacramento, California

JOHN M. McCALL, PhD, PharMac LLC
ReveraGen Biopharma, Rockville, Maryland

CRAIG M. McDONALD, MD
Professor and Chair, Department of Physical Medicine and Rehabilitation; Professor of Pediatrics; Director, NIDRR Rehabilitation Research and Training Center in Neuromuscular Diseases; Co-Director, Neuromuscular Disease Clinics, University of California Davis Health System, Sacramento, California

JERRY R. MENDELL, MD
Professor of Pediatrics and Neurology, The Ohio State University College of Medicine; Director, Center for Gene Therapy, Research Institute, Nationwide Children's Hospital, Columbus, Ohio; Director, Wellstone Muscular Dystrophy Cooperative Research Center, Rochester, New York

JORDI MIRÓ, PhD
Professor and Director, Unit for the Study and Treatment of Pain - ALGOS, Centre de Recerca en Avaluació i Mesura del Comportament, Institut d'Investigació Sanitària Pere Virgili, Universitat Rovira i Virgili, Catalonia, Spain

KANNEBOYINA NAGARAJU, DVM, PhD
Professor, Department of Integrative Systems Biology, George Washington University School of Medicine; Co-Director, Center for Genetic Medicine Research, Children's National Medical Center, Washington, DC; ReveraGen Biopharma, Rockville, Maryland

MATT OSECHECK, MA, CCC-SLP
Department of Physical Medicine and Rehabilitation, University of California Davis, Sacramento, California

BJORN OSKARSSON, MD
Director of the Multidisciplinary ALS Clinic, Assistant Professor, Department of Neurology, University of California Davis, Sacramento, California

AARON PIERCE, MS, ATP
Independent Consultant, San Diego, California

ERICA REEVES, PhD
Vice President, Research and Operations, ReveraGen Biopharma, Rockville, Maryland

DAVID RICHMAN, MD
Professor, Department of Neurology, University of California Davis, Sacramento, California

ROLANDO F. ROBERTO, MD
Associate Professor, Residency Program Director, Adult and Pediatric Spine Surgery, Department of Orthopaedic Surgery, University of California Davis, Sacramento, California

ANDREW J. SKALSKY, MD
Assistant Professor, Department of Pediatrics, University of California San Diego; Chief of Pediatric Rehabilitation Medicine, Rady Children's Hospital, San Diego, California

AMANDA E. SMITH, BS
Department of Rehabilitation Medicine, University of Washington School of Medicine, Seattle, Washington

PHILIP T. THRUSH, MD
Fellow in Pediatric Cardiology, The Heart Center, Nationwide Children's Hospital, Columbus, Ohio

GREGG K. VANDEKEIFT, MD, MA
Hospice and Palliative Care Services, Providence Health Services, Olympia, Washington

LISA F. WOLFE, MD
Associate Professor of Medicine, Division of Pulmonary and Critical Care Medicine, Northwestern University Feinberg School of Medicine, Chicago, Illinois

Contents

> In recent years nutrition assessment and management in amyotrophic lateral sclerosis (ALS) have drawn increased attention. Frequent evaluation of nutrition status is warranted in ALS, given the common occurrence of dysphagia and hypermetabolism and varying disease progression rates. Nutrition management includes dietary and swallow strategies, possible gastrostomy tube placement, and recommendations for vitamin and mineral supplementation. Strategies to assess and optimize nutrition status and prolong survival in ALS patients are reviewed with recommendations based on current research.

> This article reviews the recent literature regarding bone health as it relates to the patient living with neuromuscular disease (NMD). Studies defining the scope of bone-related disease in NMD are scant. The available evidence is discussed, focusing on abnormal calcium metabolism, increased fracture risk, and the prevalence of both scoliosis and hypovitaminosis D in Duchenne muscular dystrophy, amyotrophic lateral sclerosis, and spinal muscular atrophy. Future directions are discussed, including the urgent need for studies both to determine the nature and extent of poor bone health, and to evaluate the therapeutic effect of available osteoporosis treatments in patients with NMD.

> For generations, the neuromuscular disorder care community has focused on establishing the correct diagnosis and providing supportive care. As the pathophysiology and genetics of these conditions became better understood, novel treatments targeting the disease mechanism were developed. This has led to some significant disease-modifying and supportive treatments for several neuromuscular disorders. The current treatments for amyotrophic lateral sclerosis (ALS), neuromuscular junction disorders, inflammatory myopathies, and myotonia are reviewed. Additionally, investigational treatments for ALS, Duchenne muscular dystrophy, and spinal muscular atrophy are discussed.

Although prednisone has never been formally approved for use in Duchenne muscular dystrophy (DMD) by regulatory agencies, its efficacy has been confirmed in trials dating from the 1980s. There is a strong need for optimization of both specific type of glucocorticoid (eg, prednisone, vs deflazacort or others) and the dosing regimen. Ideally an optimized regimen would maximize efficacy while minimizing side-effect profiles. A new trial, FOR-DMD, aims to address this gap in knowledge. In parallel, there has been progress in the area of "dissociative steroids," drugs that are able to better separate efficacy and side effects, providing a broader therapeutic window.

Restrictive lung disease occurs commonly in patients with neuromuscular disease. The earliest sign of respiratory compromise in the patient with neuromuscular disease is nocturnal hypoventilation, which progresses over time to include daytime hypoventilation and eventually the need for full-time mechanical ventilation. Pulmonary function testing should be done during regular follow-up visits to identify the need for assistive respiratory equipment and initiate early noninvasive ventilation. Initiation of noninvasive ventilation can improve quality of life and prolong survival in patients with neuromuscular disease.

This article addresses the pathophysiology, diagnostic approaches, and therapeutic options in the more common forms of muscular dystrophy, especially those seen in pediatric and young adult populations. The major emphasis is on the dystrophinopathies because their treatment options are templates for those used in various other forms of dystrophy. Most patients with cardiomyopathy are treated with angiotensin-converting enzyme inhibitors or angiotensin receptor blockers, with other agents added as the disease progresses. Destination therapies and transplantation options are mentioned where appropriate. Some dystrophies can have significant conduction abnormalities requiring pacemaker treatment. Others with ventricular tachydysrhythmias may necessitate internal cardiac defibrillator placement.

Surgical management of spinal deformity in neuromuscular diseases (NMDs) often requires a multidisciplinary approach beginning in the preoperative surgical planning period, owing to concomitant restrictive lung disease and cardiomyopathy in selected NMD conditions. The need for thorough and thoughtful discussions must occur with the family and other caregivers before any scheduled surgery. The decision to proceed with spinal instrumentation may alter functional abilities in weak and marginally ambulatory NMD patients. With care and treatment involving a multidisciplinary team, proper planning, and support, patients will likely experience rewarding outcomes and improved quality of life.

Mobility-assistive technologies allow patients with neuromuscular disease to interact with peers and the community. In children, they also serve to facilitate development. Lack of access to appropriate assistive technology, especially in regards to mobility, can have adverse developmental consequences. There are multiple options for mobility devices and methods for their control. These devices can be integrated with other electronics to facilitate the control of a variety of devices in the environment. The clinician should assess which devices are best based on the patient's, caregivers', and medical team's goals.

The importance of pain extent (ie, number of body areas with pain) and pain site as factors contributing to dysfunction in persons with chronic, slowly progressive neuromuscular disease (NMD), remains poorly understood. This article discusses the importance of assessing pain site in addition to global pain intensity in patients with chronic, slowly progressive NMD. The importance of addressing pain at multiple sites will have a major impact on future studies assessing interventions to treat pain in this patient population.

This article discusses the role of palliative care in the treatment pathway of patients with progressive neuromuscular disease (NDM), including amyotrophic lateral sclerosis and Duchenne muscular dystrophy (DMD). People with severe NMDs like DMD are now living much longer, well in to adulthood. This makes them suitable for the medical model of palliative care. Yet palliative medicine is a new area, especially for "adults" with DMD. Strategies for identifying the most effective modalities to alleviate suffering in patients with an NMD receiving palliative services and creating best practice standards in pain and symptom management for this patient population are discussed.

PHYSICAL MEDICINE & REHABILITATION CLINICS OF NORTH AMERICA

NOW AVAILABLE FOR YOUR iPhone and iPad

Foreword

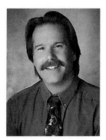

Gregory T. Carter, MD, MS
Consulting Editor

I am very excited to introduce this second volume of the *Physical Medicine and Rehabilitation Clinics of North America* on Neuromuscular Disease Management and Rehabilitation. This issue centers on "Specialty Care and Therapeutics" and is again guest edited by Drs Craig M. McDonald and Nanette C. Joyce. As with Part I of this issue, Drs McDonald and Joyce have assembled an outstanding group of authors, all of whom have contributed fantastic articles.

Dr Marlia Braun and colleagues start off with a thorough discussion of "Nutrition Assessment and Management in Amyotrophic Lateral Sclerosis," an area of tremendous importance for those of us who care for ALS patients. Many of the nutritional principles discussed here have broad applicability to other diseases as well. Dr Paula Clemens, along with Dr Joyce and Lauren P. Hache, MS, CGC, does an excellent job discussing "Bone Health and Associated Metabolic Complications in Neuromuscular Diseases," again another critical topic for this patient population. Next, an excellent update on "Current Pharmacologic Management in Selected Neuromuscular Diseases" is provided by Drs Skalsky, Oskarsson, and Richman. Dr Richman is a world-renowned expert in myasthenia and brings enormous expertise.

Speaking of enormous expertise, it is hard to overstate the expertise of Drs Eric Hoffman, Erica Reeves, Jesse Damsker, Kanneboyina Nagaraju, John M. McCall, Edward M. Connor and Kate Bushby. They provide us with a cutting-edge update on the use of corticosteroids to manage dystrophinopathies. Following that is an expert treatise on pulmonary management by Drs Wolfe, Joyce, McDonald, Benditt, and Finder. All of these authors have served the Muscular Dystrophy Association in many advisory roles and are recognized experts. Dr Benditt was just appointed to a newly formed clinical management advisory board with the MDA. An update on "Cardiac Management in Neuromuscular Diseases" is provided by an esteemed group, including Drs Allen, Thrush, Hoffman, Flanigan, and Mendell. Dr Jerry Mendell is perhaps the world's foremost expert in the management of Duchenne dystrophy. It is an honor to have him as an author here; he is in good company for sure.

The "Treatment of Spine Deformity in Neuromuscular Diseases" is nicely covered by Drs Maitra, Roberto, McDonald, and Gupta. There are some very nice illustrative radiographs provided here. The challenging task of covering "Mobility-Assistive

Phys Med Rehabil Clin N Am 23 (2012) xi–xii
http://dx.doi.org/10.1016/j.pmr.2012.08.025
1047-9651/12/$ – see front matter © 2012 Elsevier Inc. All rights reserved.

Technology in Progressive Neuromuscular Disease" was left to a very able group, including Drs Lin, Skalsky, and McDonald, along with technology expert, Aaron Pierce, MS, ATP.

The issue closes with a topic near and dear to my heart, managing chronic pain in the setting of palliative care. My esteemed colleagues, Drs Miro, Gertz, and Jensen, discuss the importance of pain site and intensity in NMD patients with chronic pain. Dr Jensen is an internationally recognized expert in the field of chronic pain and has been an enormous resource for me in terms of my own research. Last, Drs Joyce, Abresch, and VandeKeift, along with our research coordinator, Ms Smith, discuss the role of palliative care in managing progressive neuromuscular disease. Our co-author, Dr Gregg VandeKeift, has been an instrumental leader in this newly emerging field of palliative medicine.

I am so grateful to Drs McDonald and Joyce, and to each and every one of the esteemed authors here who dedicated so much time and energy to bring you this issue of the *Physical Medicine and Rehabilitation Clinics of North America*. I also want to thank our editor from Elsevier, Jessica McCool, for her patience and wisdom in helping bring this all together.

I join in with our guest editors in the dedication to Dr William M. "Bill" Fowler Jr, who was a true pioneer in the rehabilitation management of neuromuscular disease. He has been a mentor and role model for so many of us and has been a hugely positive influence on my career and my own personal and professional development.

Gregory T. Carter, MD, MS
Regional Neuromuscular Center
Providence Medical Group
410 Providence Lane, Building 2
Olympia, WA 9806, USA

E-mail address:
gtcarter@uw.edu

Despite well-documented efficacy in many chronic inflammatory conditions, chronic use of glucocorticoids also results in an extensive list of side effects, including stunting of growth, weight gain, adrenal suppression, mood changes, decreased bone density, muscle wasting and weakness, and many others. Treatment of DMD with daily prednisone was found to improve muscle strength and delay disease progression with confirmatory placebo-controlled double-blinded clinical trials occurring in the 1980s. Professor Eric Hoffman, from the Center for Genetic Medicine Research, Children's National Medical Center, Washington, DC, and colleagues review the current efforts to optimize both the specific type of glucocorticoid (eg, prednisone vs deflazacort, or others) and the dosing regimen (daily, every other day, weekend) in DMD. Dr Hoffman's group and others have made progress in the area of "dissociative steroids" — drugs that are able to separate efficacy and side effects, providing a broader therapeutic window. One such dissociative steroid, a Δ-9,11 drug, is being developed for DMD, and preclinical data suggest better optimization of the balance of efficacy and side effects.

Restrictive lung disease occurs commonly in pediatric and adult patients with neuromuscular disease. Common pediatric diseases with impaired ventilation and airway clearance include DMD and SMA types I and II. In adults, ALS is the most common NMD associated with severe pulmonary complications from neuromuscular weakness producing restrictive lung disease and clearance of airway secretions. The earliest sign of respiratory compromise in the patient with NMD is nocturnal hypoventilation, which progresses over time to include daytime hypoventilation and eventually the need for full-time mechanical ventilation. Dr Lisa Wolfe, a pulmonologist from Northwestern University in Chicago, and colleagues from both adult and pediatric pulmonary medicine and physiatry review the management of pulmonary complications in NMD with a description of many new technologies to provide noninvasive ventilation and improved pulmonary toilet. Appropriate and timely initiation of noninvasive ventilation can improve quality of life and prolong survival in patients with NMDs.

The article by Dr Hugh Allen, a pediatric cardiologist from Texas Children's Hospital and Baylor College of Medicine, and colleagues from Nationwide Children's Hospital in Columbus, Ohio addresses the cardiac manifestations, pathophysiology, and treatment of the more common forms of muscular dystrophy, especially those seen in the pediatric and young adult populations. The emphasis of this article is on the ventricular dysfunction seen in dystrophinopathies in that their treatment options are templates for those used in various other forms of dystrophy. Most cardiomyopathy patients are treated with afterload reducers such as angiotensin-converting enzyme inhibitors (ACE-I) or angiotensin receptor blockers, with the addition of other agents such as diuretics or β-blockers as the disease progresses. Emerging is the concept of destination therapies such as left ventricular assist devices and transplantation. Some of the dystrophies, such as Emery-Dreifuss or myotonic dystrophy, can have significant conduction abnormalities requiring pacemaker treatment. Others with ventricular tachydysrhythmias may necessitate internal cardiac defibrillator placement.

Dr Sukanta Maitra and colleagues from the UC Davis Health System next address the management of spinal deformity, which may adversely affect quality of life in several progressive NMDs. Severe spinal deformity in NMDs leads to poor sitting balance, pelvic obliquity, and greater likelihood of pressure sores, functional impairment, poor cosmesis, and reduced quality of life. The surgical management of spinal deformity in NMDs often requires a multidisciplinary approach beginning in the preoperative surgical planning period and continuing to the perioperative and postoperative periods, owing to concomitant restrictive lung disease and cardiomyopathy in selected NMD conditions. Such a multidisciplinary approach leads to optimal planning, prevention of complications, support of patients and families, and improved outcomes.

Dr Wendy Lin from Rady Children's Hospital and the University of California, San Diego School of Medicine, along with her colleagues, provides an informative review of the role of mobility-assistive technologies in patients with progressive NMD. Lack of appropriate access to mobility-assistive technology in children can have adverse developmental consequences. Children as young as 24 months can learn to safely operate a power wheelchair. The NMD multidisciplinary team needs to consider the patient abilities and the specific neuromuscular disease, plan for future disease progression, and provide proper and modifiable seating and positioning to maximize function and optimize the use of mobility-assistive technologies. The reduced cost of novel electronic control systems to integrate with environmental control systems and computer access makes these devices more available to a wider range of NMD patients.

Physiatrists often participate with the multidisciplinary team in the management of chronic pain syndromes in NMDs. The available data suggest that pain extent and intensity at specific sites are associated with pain interference and negatively impact physical and psychological functioning. The article by Dr Greg Carter and colleagues discusses the importance of assessing the pain site in addition to global pain intensity in patients with chronic, slowly progressive NMDs. The importance of addressing pain at multiple sites will have a major impact on future studies assessing interventions to treat pain in these patient populations. Today, there is wide recognition that the principles of palliative care should be applied as early as possible in the course of any chronic, ultimately fatal illness. This change in thinking emerged from a new understanding that problems at the end of life have their origins at an earlier time in the trajectory of disease. According to the World Health Organization definition of *palliative care*, it is an approach that improves the quality of life of patients and their families facing the problems associated with life-threatening illness, through the prevention and relief of suffering by means of early identification and accurate assessment and treatment of pain and other problems, including physical, psychosocial, and spiritual domains. The new concept of palliative care emphasizes living as well as possible with a disease. This emphasis is engendered in Dr Carter's final article, which discusses the role of palliative care in the treatment pathway of patients with progressive NMD, including ALS and DMD. People with severe NMDs like DMD and ALS are now living much longer. Strategies are discussed for identifying the most effective modalities to alleviate suffering and improve quality of life in NMD patients receiving palliative services. Best practice standards in pain and symptom management for these patient populations are discussed.

Much of our research in neuromuscular diseases over the years at UC Davis has been funded by the National Institute on Disability and Rehabilitation Research (NIDRR), the largest federal funding source for medical rehabilitation research and training. We recently received a NIDRR Advanced Rehabilitation Research Training Grant focused on training rehabilitation scientists in Neuromuscular and Neurodevelopmental Disorders. NIDRR is to be commended for their long commitment to medical rehabilitation research and research training for persons with neuromuscular diseases.

It has been encouraging to see an increase in the National Institutes of Health, Centers for Disease Control , and Department of Defense portfolios devoted to neuromuscular diseases. The situation in muscular dystrophy is a case in point. In 2001, as a result of effective lobbying efforts by a number of consumer advocacy groups such as the Muscular Dystrophy Association (MDA), Parent Project Muscular Dystrophy, FacioScapuloHumeral Muscular Dystrophy Society, Myotonic Dystrophy Foundation, and others, landmark muscular dystrophy legislation was introduced in Congress. At the time the bill, the Muscular Dystrophy Community Assistance, Research, and Education Amendments (MD-CARE Act), was unveiled in 2001, few bright spots existed for patients and families battling muscular dystrophy. Federal research for varied forms of muscular dystrophy and progressive neuromuscular diseases was minimal; surveillance and data collection were nonexistent, and the federal government lacked a comprehensive muscular dystrophy research and care agenda. The MD-CARE Act forever changed this landscape. Similar advocacy efforts by the Muscular Distrophy Association, the ALS Association, Families of SMA, Charcot-Marie-Tooth Disease Association, and many other advocacy groups are producing great awareness, improved care standards, and increased nonprofit and federal funding for a variety of other NMDs.

As mentioned in the preface in Part I of this issue, the number of MDA-sponsored neuromuscular disease clinics that have active participation by a Physical Medicine and Rehabilitation (PM&R) specialist remains a substantial minority. While over 20 Accreditation Council for Graduate Medical Education–approved Neuromuscular Medicine Fellowships have been developed in US Neurology Departments, there remains just one such training program housed in a Department of Physical Medicine and Rehabilitation (at UC Davis). Our hope is that these two issues will perhaps demonstrate the value of physiatry to current practicing Neuromuscular Medicine specialists, increase participation of PM&R specialists in NMD clinics, spur physiatry residents to consider subspecialty training in Neuromuscular Medicine, motivate the young faculty in PM&R who have graduated from our program and other Neurology-based fellowship programs to develop their own fellowship training programs in Neuromuscular Medicine, and ultimately expand the rehabilitation expertise among all Neuromuscular Medicine specialists. The ultimate goal of these two issues, focusing on diagnostic issues, therapy by allied health providers, specialty care, and disease-altering therapeutic management, is to improve the quality of life for people with neuromuscular diseases and their families.

It should be mentioned that the prior issue was dedicated to William M. Fowler Jr, MD, a pioneer in the rehabilitation management of persons with neuromuscular diseases (see Dedication in Part I). Bill Fowler continues to be a mentor to both Dr Gregory Carter, the Consulting Editor of the *PM&R Clinics*, and Dr Craig McDonald, the senior Guest Editor of these two issues. No physiatrist in history has been as instrumental as Dr Bill Fowler in advancing the scientific basis of the rehabilitation management of neuromuscular diseases.

Finally, we wish to personally thank all of the contributing authors for all the time and hard work they invested in the articles in Parts I and II, which will provide a tremendous wealth of clinical expertise that can be directly applied to your practice.

Craig M. McDonald, MD
Department of Physical Medicine and Rehabilitation
NIDRR Rehabilitation Research and Training Center
In Neuromuscular Diseases
Neuromuscular Disease Clinics
University of California Davis Health System
Sacramento, CA 95817, USA

Nanette C. Joyce, DO
Department of Physical Medicine and Rehabilitation
University of California, Davis Health System
4860 Y Street Suite 3850
Sacramento, CA 95817, USA

E-mail addresses:
craig.mcdonald@ucdmc.ucdavis.edu (C.M. McDonald)
Nanette.joyce@ucdmc.ucdavis.edu (N.C. Joyce)

Nutrition Assessment and Management in Amyotrophic Lateral Sclerosis

Marlia M. Braun, PhD, RD, CSSD[a],*, Matt Osecheck, MA, CCC-SLP[b],
Nanette C. Joyce, DO, MAS[b]

KEYWORDS

- Amyotrophic lateral sclerosis • Nutrition • Malnutrition • Gastrostomy
- Hypermetabolism • Refeeding syndrome

KEY POINTS

- Malnutrition, due to dysphagia, muscle atrophy, and hypermetabolism, in amyotrophic lateral sclerosis (ALS) is best defined as greater than 10% loss of body weight in conjunction with body mass index (BMI) less than18 kg/m^2 for 18-year-old to 65-year-old patients and BMI 20 kg/m^2 for patients greater than 65 years old. Biochemical indices for malnutrition assessment are less reliable.
- Hypermetabolism occurs in ALS patients and the cause is not yet well understood. When calculating resting energy expenditure (REE), it is estimated that an additional 10% needs to be added to standard calculations to meet the caloric needs of ALS patients.
- To accommodate changes in swallowing and chewing, soft, moist, and thickened foods served chilled are recommended. Hydration needs to be monitored closely. Speech therapy can provide instruction on safe practices to reduce aspiration and choking risk.
- Placement of a radiologically inserted gastrostomy (RIG) tube may confer safety advantages over a percutaneous endoscopic gastrostomy (PEG), but there is controversy as to whether a feeding tube in general improves survival rate. Consideration for and placement of a gastrostomy tube should occur early and recommendations suggest placing the tube before forced vital capacity (FVC) drops below 50% predicted values.
- Complications during refeeding after gastrostomy tube placement have not been studied in the ALS population but should be given consideration when initiating tube feeding.

[a] Department of Food and Nutrition Services, University of California Davis, 2315 Stockton Boulevard, Sacramento, CA 95817, USA; [b] Department of Physical Medicine and Rehabilitation, University of California Davis, 4860 Y Street, Suite 3850, Sacramento, CA 95817, USA
* Corresponding author.
E-mail address: marlia.braun@ucdmc.ucdavis.edu

Phys Med Rehabil Clin N Am 23 (2012) 751–771
http://dx.doi.org/10.1016/j.pmr.2012.08.006
1047-9651/12/$ – see front matter © 2012 Elsevier Inc. All rights reserved.

INTRODUCTION

ALS is a complex neurodegenerative disease that results in the progressive loss of both upper and lower motor neurons, causing rapidly progressive disability from paralysis of skeletal muscles. ALS is inevitably fatal and the one Food and Drug Administration–approved disease-modifying medication, Rilutek (Riluzole), prolongs life modestly by only months without significant impact on function or quality of life. Therapies addressing symptomatic complaints continue to provide the mainstay of care for patients with ALS. Some of these palliative treatments provide survival benefits beyond that achieved with disease-modifying medication.

Over the past 15 years, the literature regarding the nutritional needs of patients with ALS and how weight and calorie balance influence disease progression and survival has grown, becoming more notable and significant. In addition to loss in motor neuron function having an impact on calorie and fluid intake by impairing swallow and shifting percentage lean tissue mass from skeletal muscle atrophy, these patients also, surprisingly, present with hypermetabolism. The metabolic basis for this hypermetabolism has not been fully elucidated, but this syndrome, which often accompanies ALS, further complicates patients' nutritional status from an energy balance standpoint, placing them at high risk for malnutrition. This has necessarily resulted in recommendations to more closely and carefully follow and then individualize nutrition assessment and management to optimize quality and length of life. The most impactful nutritional issues for these patients include dysphagia, hypophagia, dehydration, weight loss, the consideration and timing of placement of a gastrostomy (PEG) tube, and, if a gastrostomy tube is placed, the potential for refeeding syndrome (RFS) as adequate nutritional support is initiated.

NUTRITION ASSESSMENT
Malnutrition

Malnutrition is described as loss of greater than 10% of body weight or a BMI lower than 18.5 kg/m^2, and both are considered negative predictors of survival in ALS patients. The prevalence of malnutrition in the ALS population varies among reports, from 16% to 53%.[1] Malnutrition can initiate a vicious cycle for ALS patients, further compromising muscle strength[2] and respiratory capacity due to weakening of both skeletal and respiratory muscles[3] beyond that caused by motor neuron loss. The literature overwhelming shows that a low BMI and malnutrition negatively affect disease progression and thus the survival in ALS patients. Malnourished ALS patients have a 7.7-fold increased risk in mortality.[4–7]

Anthropometrics

Malnutrition can be assessed using various methods, including anthropometric data, such as body weight, BMI, triceps skinfold thickness (TSF), and midarm muscle circumference (MAMC).[8] It is believed that a sheer reduction in body weight of 5% to 10% from normal can suggest compromised nutritional status and be a prognostic factor for survival.[9–11] Unfortunately, this range has not been validated in ALS patients. Studies have shown, however, BMI to be strongly associated with survival in ALS with malnutrition below 18.5 kg/m^2 for all ages or less than 18.5 kg/m^2 for ages 18 to 65 and below 20 kg/m^2 for patients over 65 years old.[12] A retrospective study of 427 ALS patients found a U-shaped relationship between BMI and survival with maximum survival observed in patients with BMI of 30 to 35, even when adjusting for FVC, bulbar onset, use of Rilutek, and duration of the disease.[13] Paganoni and colleagues[13] found patients with BMI greater than 35 had greater mortality due to higher frequency of cardiovascular disease (which was also a significant predictor of survival). The use of BMI, however, as a reliable assessment tool for the ALS population is questionable due to neurogenic atrophy, energy imbalance, and dependent edema caused by immobility.

Height and weight measurements are useful; however, they do not give information regarding the type of tissue gained or lost with changes in body weight. Changes in body composition can be assessed using other tools, such as TSF, which provide data regarding fat mass that can be followed over time. TSF is measured using Harpenden calipers, and these measures are compared with a reference table to determine leanness or excessive body fat.[14] Unfortunately, fat distribution is not even; therefore, measuring skinfolds at multiple sites is believed to improve the accuracy of the assessment although no consensus exists as to which combination of sites is best for accurate measurement.[15]

Additionally, there are tools designed to assess somatic protein (skeletal protein mass), which is the body's major protein store and can be used to assess malnutrition.[16] Measuring somatic protein using the following techniques can be used to track protein nutritional status and be quanitified using standardized tables by gender and age. MAMC gives information about lean body mass using TSF and midarm circumference (MAC) in a formula.[8] The clinical status of ALS patients has been monitored using bone-free arm muscle area (AMA), which combines the TSF and MAMC measurements (**Box 1**).[17] AMA has been used for studies in the ALS population, providing serial assessment of muscle atrophy. AMA measures correlated significantly with body mass, FVC, and maximal voluntary ventilation.[4,18] These measures are limited, however, in ALS due to upper limb dysfunction and muscle wasting. Despite their ease of use, the results from ALS patients compared with reference tables may not accurately depict patients' nutrition status.

Body Composition

Body composition, the assessment of body fat and FFM, can additionally be used to track changes as the disease progresses. Various techniques can be used to measure body composition and each varies in cost and portability. A portable, inexpensive, and simple procedure is bioelectrical impedance analysis (BIA). BIA uses electrical current to measure resistance of body compartments to establish values for lean body mass, fat mass, and total body water.

There are 3 types of devices, 500 kHz monofrequency and 50-kHz and 100-kHz dual-frequency and multifrequency BIAs. BIA has been used in several ALS studies.[4,7,12] In 2003, BIA was validated as an outcome measure for ALS studies for both longitudinal tracking and single examination measurements with the use of an adapted equation in conjunction with a frequency of 50 kHz.[19]

Box 1
Somatic protein assessments

MAMC[8]

　　MAMC = MAC (cm) − 0.314 × TSF (mm)

AMA[17]

　　Men: [(MAC − pi × TSF)^2/4 pi] − 10 cm^2

　　Women: [(MAC − pi × TSF)^2/4 pi] − 6.5 cm^2

π = 3.14.

Dual-energy x-ray absorptiometry (DXA) directly measures the body's absorption of x-rays at 2 energy levels, which allows for the direct measurement of body compartments.[20] It is more expensive to use and less portable than BIA. DXA has been used as a measure in the ALS population and studies have found a reduction in fat mass, muscle mass, and bone mass with a fat mass/muscle mass ratio that was low or normal compared with myogenic atrophy patients and control patients. Kanda and colleagues[20] additionally found that DXA provided a clearer distinction between myogenic atrophy and neurogenic atrophy due to increased fat infiltration in the myogenic atrophied skeletal muscle. DXA has provided confirmatory data that ALS patients lose lean body mass over time despite normal or elevated calorie intake.[21] Therefore, weight maintenance or gain in this population, as disease progresses, is likely a reflection of change in body composition with an increase in fat stores. In another study by Tandan and colleagues[22] that followed patients over 1 year, reduced lean body mass occurred over time that correlated with the ALS functional rating scale but not with total body weight, BMI, or FVC.

Both of these tools, BIA and DXA, can track body composition change over time, but each presents a different challenge related to cost, availability, and patient comfort. No definitive studies using either BIA or DXA have demonstrated that the observed changes in tissue distribution are a prognostic factor for survival.[4] It has been argued, however, that a higher fat mass is beneficial for survival in the ALS population[11,23] due to an observed progressive reduction in body fat stores associated with proximity to death.[4] Additionally, knowledge of a patient's fat-free mass (FFM) weight, as determined by BIA or DXA, can assist in estimating energy needs in relation to ALS-associated hypermetabolism (discussed later).

Biochemical Indices

Serum markers are useful for different purposes when assessing the nutritional status of ALS patients. Certain serum markers provide information regarding the current nutritional state of patients, whereas others correlate with disease progression and survival. Serum markers used for the assessment of malnutrition in ALS patients include serum albumin, prealbumin, hemoglobin, magnesium, calcium (total and ionized), phosphorous, serum zinc and copper, and retinol-binding protein whereas the creatinine height index (CHI) has been used as a marker of disease progression and survival. CHI is a ratio of a patient's 24-hour creatinine excretion and the expected normal creatinine excretion for a given height. CHI has been shown to correlate with the degree of muscle depletion in ALS patients. A drop in CHI, with a corresponding elevation in serum calcium, has been observed in close proximity to death in ALS patients.[4] The other markers remain within normal limits, with no gender differences or changes related to time to death.[4]

These tests have been validated as markers of nutritional status in other disease populations but have not been well researched in ALS. Furthermore, these values can be altered by hydration status, inflammation, hepatic failure, or catabolism at the level of the muscle and intestine,[24] and the body often compensates to maintain normal values with slowly progressive malnutrition. Other micronutrients, such as B vitamins, vitamin D, antioxidant vitamins, and minerals, have not been well researched due to the poor correlation of blood values with intracellular stores. Thus, biochemical markers used to assess malnutrition are often less reliable then anthropometric assessments, such as monitoring body weight, BMI, and FFM.

Studies have suggested a positive correlation of hyperlipidemia and diabetes mellitus type 2 in relation to ALS disease onset and prolonged survival time. Hyperlipidemia, obesity, and diabetes mellitus type 2 were found in one study to possibly delay the onset of motor symptoms.[25] Multiple studies evaluating more than 300 subjects have found that patients with hyperlipidemia and elevated fasting total cholesterol and triglycerides as well as elevated low-density lipoprotein (LDL)/high-density lipoprotein (HDL) ratio had significantly increased survival by nearly 12 months[26–28] compared with subjects with normal serum lipid levels. Additionally, low levels of LDL and total cholesterol have been associated with lower percent pre-dicted FVC.[28] In a cross-sectional study by Ikeda and colleagues,[29] an inverse rela-tionship was observed between both total cholesterol and LDL values, when compared to the annual decline of the ALS functional rating scale and FVC.

Contrary to these findings, an earlier study of more than 600 subjects found the exact opposite, with no correlation in lipid values with survival time. The investigators observed a significant decrease in lipid levels in those patients with an FVC of less than 70% predicted and interpreted this finding as a indicator that respiratory impairment is related to a decrease in blood lipids.[30] Another study similarly found no changes in length of survival in patients with hyperlipidemia compared with patients with normal lipid values.[31] It has been argued that BMI may be a confounding factor when evalu-ating the effects of lipid levels in ALS.[31] In 427 ALS patients from 3 clinical trials assessing serum lipids, the LDL/HDL ratio was shown to not be associated with survival after adjusting for BMI.[13] As discussed previously, higher BMIs, between 30 and 35, have been associated with longer survival time in ALS. In spite of the contro-versy, changes in lipid metabolism with lowering of serum lipid levels is considered one possible sign consistent with hypermetabolism in ALS and may be a sufficient argument against the appropriateness of statin use in this population.[32–34]

Other biochemical indices studied include uric acid levels. High uric acid levels have been previously linked to a reduced risk of developing Parkinson disease and slower rates of decline as well as slower progression in Huntington disease, multiple system atrophy, and mild cognitive impairment. The mechanism remains unclear but the theory involves its antioxidant properties and its protective influence on neuronal cell death.[35–37] There have been a few studies showing reduced uric acid levels in the ALS population in comparison with healthy controls and one study found higher baseline uric acid values associated with increased survival in men with levels of 4.8 mg/dL or greater. These same uric acid levels, however, did not show an increase survival for women and only 22% had a level greater than 4.8 mg/dL.[38] Uric acid levels are notoriously higher in men than women complicating the utility of this serum marker.

Often the relevance of common biochemical indices associated with malnutrition in ALS is of questionable value and should be assessed in conjunction with anthropo-metric measurements. Biomarker research is ongoing and will uncover more accurate and reliable indices to assess nutrition status in patients with ALS. Two recent cross-sectional studies found 23 metabolites related to neuronal change, hypermetabolism, oxidative damage, and mitochondrial dysfunction that were significantly altered in plasma from ALS patients compared with healthy volunteers.[39]

Hypermetabolism

Most ALS patients suffer from hypermetabolism. Reports suggest nearly 100% of patients with familial ALS and 52% of patients with sporadic ALS[40] suffer from hyper-metabolism. Hypermetabolism is a strange paradoxic occurrence in the ALS popula-tion given denervation, reduced physical activity, and muscle atrophy. It is expected that energy requirements decline under these circumstances. This phenomenon, in conjunction with poor energy intake and swallowing difficulties, is an additional contributor to malnutrition and poor survival in the ALS population.

Hypermetabolism has most commonly been confirmed using the ratio of measured REE (mREE) to calculated REE (cREE). Findings in the ALS population often reveal a ratio greater than 1.1, or 110% of normal. The mREE is obtained by calorimetry whereas cREE is calculated using an established energy equation. Calorimetry is a measurement of the amount of heat eliminated or stored in a system. Direct calorimetry is the measurement of the amount of heat produced by a patient while housed for a certain amount of time within a small chamber. Access to equipment allowing direct calorimetry measurement is limited and often impractical.

Indirect calorimetry is a more often used measure of energy expenditure. This technique uses gas exchange measurements, oxygen consumption, and CO_2 output to determine the amount of heat produced by patients indirectly.[40] Patients are typically evaluated in a seated position for 20 to 30 minutes and asked to breathe normally under a transparent canopy. Indirect calorimetry is noninvasive and simple to perform but not regularly used to due the cost, availability of equipment, and patient tolerance. Ultimately, indirect calorimetry can be used to help assess energy expenditure and allow for customized recommendations for nutritional support to meet a patient's mREE and minimize weight loss.

Many studies have evaluated ALS patients comparing indirect calorimetry with calculated energy expenditure equations. The Harris-Benedict and the Mifflin–St Jeor equations[41] have both been recommended for use when estimating energy requirements for ALS patients (**Box 2**).[42] The Harris-Benedict equation[43] is the most commonly used in these comparison studies, which have found an increase in mREE on average of 14% to 20% beyond that predicted by the Harris-Benedict–derived cREE.[6,44,45] One study reported using the Harris-Benedict equation and overestimating patient needs; however, the study cohort included patients with mechanical ventilation, and 11 of the 34 had not fasted overnight before indirect calorimetry testing. Both of these factors compromise the data and thus the interpretation of results.[46] Current thinking supports the addition of a 10% increase in calories beyond the cREE values[42,47] when providing nutritional recommendations for patients with ALS.

The mREE represents the energy requirement necessary for homeostasis of normal bodily functions, including the cardiorespiratory, cerebral, and nervous systems as well as biochemical reactions to sustain organ function. It does not include the energy expenditure associated with physical activity or that due to the thermic effect of food. The most metabolically active tissues are the FFM, viscera, and muscle tissue. Visceral organs are responsible for 70% to 80% of the daily REE in comparison to 22% by muscle mass. In ALS, it might be assumed that resultant muscle atrophy, and reduced calorie intake, with its related reduction from the thermic effect of food, would result in decreased mREE. This is not the case, however.

Box 2
Equations for calculating resting energy expenditure in kilocalories per day

Harris-Benedict equation[43]

　Men: REE = 66.47 + 13.75 (W) + 5 (H) – 6.76 (A)

　Women: REE = 655.1 + 9.56 (W) + 1.7 (H) – 4.7 (A)

Mifflin–St Jeor equation[41]

　Men: REE = (9.99 × W) + (6.25 × H) – (4.92 × A) + 5

　Women: REE = (9.99 × W) + (6.25 × H) – (4.92 × A) – 161

W is body weight in kilograms (kg), H is height in centimeters (cm), and A is age in years.

Each organ has its own energy expenditure rate that is dependent on its weight.[48] As muscle mass is lost in an ALS patient, the patient's proportion of organ mass to muscle mass increases, shifting caloric needs due to greater calories required per kilogram of FFM.[49,50] Given this shift, there have been REE equations derived for use in ALS, adjusting for these changes in FFM, using 34 kcal/kg to 35 kcal/kg of FFM.[42,45,47,50,51] When indirect calorimetry is not available, these energy equations can be used to predict energy requirements (cREE) with expected error of approximately 150 to 250 calories.[49]

It has been argued that mREE can be used as a prognostic factor for survival. Measured REE has been followed longitudinally through the course of disease, with REE levels remaining high until the late terminal stage of disease, when a decrease is observed in mREE just before death.[44] Measured REE has been positively correlated with BMI, FFM, energy, protein intakes, and albumin levels.[44,45] The mREE has been shown to remain higher than calculated with a slight decrease at proximity of death whereas FFM remained stable.[44] This suggests REE is a prognostic factor for survival. mREE and mREE/cREE, however, have shown stable despite deterioration of the disease,[45] thus making mREE questionable as a predictor of survival. For hypermetabolism to occur in the ALS population while in the midst of decreasing physical activity and increased denervation with muscle atrophy necessarily suggests the presence of an underlying metabolic derangement.

Several hypotheses have been developed to explain the increase in mREE. One proposed mechanism is that the increased work required for functional skeletal and respiratory muscles activity in the setting of progressive loss caused by denervation results in increased energy expenditure.[4,52] Another proposed mechanism is termed, the respiratory hypothesis—that increased mREE is due to increased respiratory muscular expenditures.[4] The respiratory hypothesis seems an inadequate explanation because FVC has not been associated with mREE,[47] and although FVC decreases with disease progression and proximity to death, mREE/cREE and mREE remain stable.[4]

In addition, it has been postulated that fasciculations, spasticity, or both contribute to hypermetabolism because they theoretically increase basic muscular tone and thus REE. No correlation between fasciculation or spasticity and REE,[47] however, has been identified. Genetics may play a role in hypermetabolism because familial ALS patients consistently have higher mREE compared with sporadic ALS patients.[51] But the biologic mechanism responsible for this difference remains unknown. Lastly, the increased proportion of calorically demanding visceral tissue in the setting of reduced metabolically active muscle tissue may contribute to hypermetabolism because these organs can become metabolic sinks.

Animal models of ALS, in particular mutant SOD1 and TDP-43 mice, have contributed to understanding of ALS and its pathologic processes.[53] Both models have provided evidence in support of the hypothesis that abnormalities in muscle energy metabolism and mitochondrial function create the energy deficit and hypermetabolism seen in ALS.[54–56] Animal studies evaluating energy dysmetabolism in ALS have identified defects involving decreased production of ATP,[57,58] expression of mitochondrial uncoupling proteins, increased concentrations of markers of carbohydrate and lipid metabolism,[58,59] unspecified mitochondrial defect,[60–63] and mutant gene expression in muscle[64] and nonmuscle tissues.[65]

Further research is needed to determine the role of each of these potential contributors. ALS murine models, however, have convincingly shown that energy metabolism is impaired and is likely a major factor in creating the hypermetabolism observed in ALS patients.[66]

Muscle Atrophy, Dysphagia, and Their Influence on Nutrition

Muscle mass and contractility are dependent on chemical stimulation from motor neurons. The loss of motor neurons and associated neuromuscular junctions in ALS reduce neuronal signaling to the muscle,[67] leading to mitochondrial dysfunction with mishandling of calcium.[68] The mishandling of calcium in turn leads to the initiation of denervation-induced muscle atrophy,[69] which is further complicated by the altered function of mitochondria, resulting in increased production of reactive oxygen species and overall oxidative stress.[70] The increased oxidative stress can potentiate further muscle atrophy through muscle cell apoptosis[71,72] and muscle protein degradation.[70]

As ALS progresses, denervation of muscle tissue spreads beyond the region of first symptom, to affect other regions of the body. In spinal-onset ALS, muscle atrophy begins in the upper and/or lower limbs, eventually having an impact on a patient's ability to self-feed and maintain a seated position with head upright to facilitate a good swallow. The time it takes to independently complete a meal increases in parallel to a patient's increasing disability. Eventually, ALS patients become dependent on caregivers for feeding, which often results in further reduction of intake from early cessation of meals in an attempt by patients to avoid caregiver burden. Bulbar-onset ALS, affecting the muscles of the tongue, oropharynx, and mastication, creates nutritional challenges for patients due to progressive impairment of chewing and swallowing with resultant dysphagia. In all cases of ALS, inadequate nutrition, whatever the cause, has the potential to worsen muscle atrophy.[5,73]

Dysphagia, or difficulty swallowing, is a major cause of malnutrition in ALS patients. In cases of bulbar ALS, dysphagia can result from the involvement of the trigeminal, facial, hypoglossal, glossopharyngeal, or vagus cranial nerves.[74–76] In the early stages of ALS associated dysphagia, lingual dysfunction results in poor food bolus control, uncontrolled loss of the bolus over the back of the tongue, and delayed transition of the bolus from the oral cavity to the pharynx. In the later stages of disease, the mechanisms that cause dysphagia expand to include impaired constriction of the pharynx and decreased elevation of the larynx, resulting in bolus residue in the pyriform sinuses.[77,78] These complications, compounded by ALS patients' declining respiratory status, place these individuals at high risk for aspiration and nutritional compromise.

Dysphagia is present in 45% of patients with bulbar onset at diagnosis, and irrespective of onset, nearly 81% of all ALS patients experience dysphagia.[79] Bulbar-onset disease progresses more rapidly to dysphagia compared with spinal onset, which develops later and more slowly.[80] These statistics emphasize the importance of having a speech therapist as a member of a multidisciplinary team or available to provide care for ALS patients.

There are several techniques available to evaluate swallow function, ranging from a simple test of observing patients consume water and assessing for salivary pooling, dysarthria,[81] or speech[82] abnormalities to more complex evaluations that include the use of modalities, such as videofluoroscopy[5,83] and flexible fiberoptic laryngoscopy.[84] Patients should be asked at each regularly scheduled follow-up evaluation if they are having problems swallowing, have experienced choking episodes, or are coughing while drinking thin liquids, such as water or coffee—often the earliest sign of dysphagia. If symptoms are present, a formal evaluation by a speech therapist should be performed, a referral placed for an evaluation by a registered dietician, and conversations should begin addressing the use of gastrostomy tube in ALS. Early conversation regarding this simple procedure allows patients time to adjust to the idea of having a gastrostomy tube inserted before their swallowing and respiratory status become too impaired. These delayed and weakened oral activities ultimately result in reduced calorie and fluid intake for fear of coughing or choking and/or because of the length of time it takes to complete a meal.[7] Over time and without intervention, dysphagia in ALS patients often results in dehydration, weight loss, and malnutrition.

Dietary Recall and Dietary Modifications

A 24-hour dietary recall and dietary logs are useful tools[4,9] for registered dietitians and speech therapists. The information gathered through interviews can allow for assessment of progressive changes in dysphagia and overall intake over time. It can be a struggle, however, for patients to provide this information depending on their communication status and familiarity with quantification of portion size. It is not uncommon for overestimation to occur. Gathering of information, such as foods that trigger choking, foods that a patient purposefully avoids, and foods that are difficult to swallow, however, can be ascertained. Determining the length it takes for a typical meal and relating it to a patient's fatigue can also provide important information regarding calorie intake and hydration[85] because some patients require at least 60 minutes to consume adequate calories during a meal.[4]

Dysphagic patients often benefit from calorie dense foods to help reduce total volume necessary for adequate intake,[9,76,86] especially given the trend of mild to moderate energy deficiency.[4] Many ALS patients have been found to consume only 70% of the recommended dietary allowance for energy.[4,9] Often patients focus on consumption of a high-protein diet[4] because they believe this may ameliorate the reduction of muscle mass due to atrophy. High-energy diets, however, with more calories coming from fat to support fat stores, have been shown to modify energy metabolism, reverse expression of markers associated with muscle denervation, and reduce weight loss, all important for survival in ALS patients.[11,59,87–89]

To accommodate changes in swallowing and chewing and to avoid choking and aspiration, soft, moist, and thickened foods are often recommended.[76] Additives are available that increase the viscosity of beverages and there are beverages that are naturally thicker or prethickened commercially for use. Some supplemental nutrition drinks served chilled are thicker than if served warm or at room temperature. ALS patients benefit from proper instruction provided by a speech therapist on postures that improve swallowing[76,85,90] and reduce aspiration risk.

Constipation is a common problem due primarily to a low-fiber diet, dehydration, and minimal physical activity.[76,90] Unfortunately, this can further contribute to poor appetite.[91] Extra fluids and a mild laxative should be offered.[76,90] At some point, however, these recommendations no longer support adequate calorie intake because the dysphagia becomes so severe that the need for enteral nutrition becomes the next step.

ENTERAL NUTRITION
Percutaneous Endoscopic Gastrostomy or Radiologically Inserted Gastrostomy

When ALS patients lose more than 10% of their baseline body weight, a gastrostomy tube is often indicated. ALS patients with greater than 20% weight loss were shown to have reduced survival post–gastrostomy tube placement by 149 days compared with a group with 0% to 20% weight loss.[92] Additional indications for the placement of a gastrostomy tube include[93,94]

- Poor dietary intake related to increased length of meals, fatigue with eating, anxiety with eating, and sialorrhea
- Dehydration

- Bulbar symptoms
- Significant dysphagia with evidence of aspiration
- Declining respiratory status

Argued advantages for gastrostomy tube placement include alleviation of patient and family stress, improvement in quality of life, and increased survival.[95,96]

A gastrostomy tube is typically inserted using 1 of 2 methods. PEG has been the predominant method for gastrostomy tube placement in ALS patients presenting with minor bulbar symptoms and without significant respiratory muscle weakness, defined as FVC less than 50% of predicted values. PEG placement requires moderate sedation, use of an endoscope, and patients positioned in a recumbent position during the procedure. Hospitalization for up to 5 days after the procedure is typical. RIG placement does not require sedation or an endoscope and patients may remain in the upright position. These differences are important to consider for ALS patients with questionable respiratory function. An RIG can be placed safely in patients with an FVC of less than 50% and those using noninvasive ventilation, such as a bilevel positive airway pressure. The RIG requires an experienced interventional radiologist who inserts a nasogastric tube into the stomach to inflate it with air. Under a local anesthetic, a guide cannula for the feeding tube is introduced and secured spanning from the stomach to the abdominal wall. Patients remain in the hospital for 1 to 4 days postplacement for monitoring. With both an PEG and RIG, the use of the gastrostomy tube is typically commenced the night of the procedure, and patients are monitored for local infection.[97]

More studies are needed to determine if there is an advantage of one procedure over the other in this population. It has been argued that there is no difference in survival rate comparing the procedures.[92,97–99] Chio and colleagues, however,[100] followed 50 ALS patients with FVC less than 50% placed with either an RIG or PEG. The investigators reported a mean survival time of 204 days after RIG compared with 85 days in the PEG-treated cohort, and the respiratory function decreased more in the PEG-treated cohort. The investigators concluded that RIG was safer than PEG, especially if a patient had moderate or severe respiratory impairment.

The dilemma with gastrostomy tube initiation is the lack of definitive evidence showing improved quality of life and/or prolonged survival in the ALS population post-placement.[96] There have been many studies measuring mortality rate postprocedure, with respiratory insufficiency the most common cause of death.[101] Procedure-related mortality has been shown to be 1.8% with a 24-hour in-hospital mortality rate of 3.6% and 30-day mortality rate of 11.5%.[102] In a longitudinal study of patients post–PEG placement, survival time was 211 days to 28 months, but was not considered significantly different from non–PEG-treated patients.[103–105] Another study of 35 ALS patients with FVC greater than 50% predicted assessed patients every 3 months post–PEG tube placement for up to 2 years. The data revealed a mortality rate that did not differ significantly between patients with a PEG and those without a PEG at the 6-month mark. After 6 months, however, the mortality rate was lower in the PEG group. Additionally, the treated patients had significant improvement in BMI.[10] Contrary to these findings, a Scottish study observed a median survival rate after PEG insertion of 146 days with 1-month mortality of 25% and the PEG did not provide a survival advantage compared with those patients without a gastrostomy tube.[106] The study found spinal-onset ALS patients might have poorer survival than bulbar-onset patients post-procedure, suggesting the possibility that phenotype may influence outcome.[106]

The purpose of placing a feeding tube is to reduce dehydration, improve malnutrition in a hypermetabolic state, and stabilize weight loss with the hopes of improved survival. The literature, as reviewed previously, shows inconsistent results concerning survival rate, but many studies demonstrate weight stabilization, which by itself can contribute to prolonged survival.[5,98,100,101,107,108] Given these data, recommendations have been made that gastrostomy tube should be considered when oral intake is impaired and then placed before the FVC falls below 50% predicted.[109,110] Many patients fear a gastrostomy tube being noticeable and benefit from seeing examples showing the size and discreteness. Unfortunately, the rate of disease progression in ALS is variable and attempting to capture a patient with FVC greater than 50% predicted, who has not lost greater than 20% of body weight, and who has only mild to moderate dysphagia and is psychologically ready for the placement of a feeding tube is at times difficult.

Enteral Supplements

After a gastrostomy tube is placed and is ready for feeding initiation, the type of enteral formula used is important to consider. At this time, there are no ALS specific enteral formulas, and guidelines do not exist for artificial nutrition in ALS patients. To tackle constipation, a high-fiber formula may be appropriate, but these formulas often require extra fluid boluses to meet daily fluid requirements and reduce constipation.[111] This may require too much fluid volume and can be uncomfortable for patients. Additionally, a high-fiber formula may not provide adequate calorie needs in this hypermetabolic population.

It has been postulated that an ideal disease-specific enteral formula for the ALS population is calorically dense to reduce volume and infusion time with 1.5 or more calories per milliliter, high in fat and low in carbohydrates to minimize carbon dioxide production and possibly slow disease progression, high in omega-3 fatty acids for their anti-inflammatory properties, and high in antioxidants to combat oxidative stress in addition to being high in fiber to reduce constipation.[73] Such a formula does not exist but there are formulas targeting acute lung injury and/or acute respiratory failure that are enriched in omega-3 fats and antioxidants,[112–115] which may confer a benefit for ALS patients. Assessing the effectiveness of specific formulas on disease progression in ALS is an area of much needed research.

Refeeding Syndrome

With the initiation of enteral feeding in a population suffering from malnutrition, consideration must be given and treatment provided to avoid RFS. RFS typically occurs when patients are fed after a period of starvation. The underlying causes include fluid, electrolyte, and hormonal imbalances,[116,117] as described in **Table 1**. Such changes can adversely affect cardiac, respiratory, hematologic, hepatic, and neuromuscular systems, leading to clinical complications and, at their most severe, death. The incidence and severity of RFS have not been studied in ALS.

With prolonged and severe malnutrition, the gut mucosa can atrophy and pancreatic insufficiency develops, resulting in diarrhea once initiation of enteral nutrition has occurred, which further amplifies electrolyte and mineral imbalances. The National Institute for Health and Clinical Excellence (NICE) has created guidelines for determining patients at high risk for developing RFS[118] (**Table 2**).[116] The characteristics of patients at high risk for RFS are commonly seen in ALS patients.

RFS prevention is the key to treatment in the outpatient setting due to the lack of access to laboratory and hospital monitoring. The nadir for RFS usually occurs within the first 5 days after initiation of enteral feeding. Most patients have already been discharged from the hospital after gastrostomy placement at this time and are home without surveillance. Signs and symptoms that commonly occur with refeeding

Table 1
Dietary supplements and their targeted therapy

Oxidative stress	Selenium, vitamin D, vitamin A, vitamin E, carotenoids, folate, vitamin B_{12}, vitamin B_6, corcumin, ginseng, glutathione, phytoestrogens, α-lipoic acid, grape seed extract, pycnogenol, coenzyme Q10, ginkgo biloba, green tea, NAC, MAK, epigallocatechin gallate, L-carnitine, melatonin
Antiglutamatergic	DHEA, phytoestrogens, lipoic acid, grape seed extract, pycnogenol, branched-chain amino acids, magnesium
Mitochondrial dysfunction	Coenzyme Q10, carnitine, creatine monohydrate, pyruvate
Mutant SOD1 stabilization	Copper chelators, ascorbate, zinc

DHEA: dehydroepiandrosterone; NAC: N-acetylcysteine; MAK: Maharishi amrit kalesh.
Data from Refs.[23,126,127]

include abdominal pain, constipation, vomiting, muscle weakness, dyspnea, delirium, tremors, parasthesias, and hyperglycemia.[119] Strategies used to avoid RFS involve vitamin and nutrient supplementation before gastrostomy tube placement and should be continued during the initiation of enteral feeding. Patients should be instructed to take the following supplements for at least 10 days before gastrostomy tube placement[117–119]:

- Thiamine: 200–300 mg daily
- Vitamin B_{12}: 2.4 μg 1–2 times daily
- Vitamin B_6: 1.7 mg daily
- Folate: 400 μg daily, not to exceed 1 mg daily
- Selenium: 20–70 μg daily
- Zinc: 2.5–5 mg daily
- Iron: 10–15 mg daily

Guidelines for the initiation of enteral formula begin with delivery of 10 kcal/kg on day 1 with cases of extreme malnutrition starting with only 5 kcal/kg. On days 2

Table 2
Refeeding syndrome characteristics

Salt and water retention	Carbohydrate intake results in reduced renal excretion of sodium and water causing edema and possible heart failure
Hypokalemia	Related to insulin secretion, resulting in rapid uptake of potassium into cells as glucose and amino acids are absorbed for glycogen and protein synthesis
Hypophosphatemia	Important intracellular mineral needed for increased phosphorylation of glucose, ATP production, and control for the affinity of the oxygen binding to hemoglobin
Thiamine deficiency	Is a cofactor in glycolysis with deficiency leading to Korsakoff syndrome, Wernike encephalopathy, and/or cardiomyopathy
Hypomagnesemia	Rapid carbohydrate loading after starvation causes rapid cellular uptake. Magnesium is an important co-factor in most enzyme systems, including oxidative phosphorylation and ATP production

Data from Stanga Z, Brunner A, et al. Nutrition in clinical practice-the refeeding syndrome: illustrative cases and guidelines for prevention and treatment. Eur J Clin Nutr 2008;62(6):687–94; and Mehanna H, Nankivell PC, Moledina J, et al. Refeeding syndrome—awareness, prevention and management. Head Neck Oncol 2009;1:4.

through 4, enteral feeding can be increased by a maximum of 5 kcal/kg/d, assuring patient tolerance. By days 5 through 7, increases of 20 kcal/kg/d to 30 kcal/kg/d can be provided with further increases at day 8 and beyond, depending on a patient's goal. During this first week, patients may need to restrict added fluids to avoid hyponatremia.[117–120] In the meantime, patients and caregivers should be instructed to monitor for signs and symptoms of RFS and seek medical care should they occur.

In a perfect setting, laboratory values would be followed over 8 days with adjustments made to provide necessary electrolytes and nutrients by intravenous administration. Some serum electrolyte values, in particular magnesium, are resistant to changes in the serum even as malnutrition progresses[121–123] and it should be assumed that changes have occurred when greater than 10% of body weight has been lost.[124] In the home setting, patients should complete their 10-day course of supplementation and then rely on a daily multivitamin with trace minerals in addition to the micronutrients provided by the formula. Efforts should be made to provide these supplements in a form that patients can successfully manage even in the case of severe dysphagia. Once a gastrostomy tube has been placed, supplements can be crushed and put through the feeding tube with water.

RFS has been studied in many conditions, including cancer, anorexia, chronic alcoholism, malabsorptive states, prolonged fasting, and dysphagia, among others,[119] but has yet to be studied in the ALS population. Many ALS patients are at risk according to the NICE criteria (**Box 3**).[118] Prophylactic supplementation may reduce mortality rates related to feeding tube placement and prolong survival in this patient population.

SUPPLEMENTS

Hypotheses related to the pathophysiology of ALS onset and progression include oxidative damage, mitochondrial dysfunction, inflammation, glutamate excitotoxicity, and protein and RNA toxicity due to genetic mutations, among others. In an effort to combat the biologic effects that cause disease or promote its progression, the use of dietary supplements has been proposed and explored and a few such as creatinine

---

Box 3
NICE criteria for patients at high risk for developing refeeding problems

Patient has 1 or more of the following:

- BMI less than 16 kg/m^2

- Unintentional weight loss of greater than 15% within the previous 3–6 months

- Little or no nutritional intake for more than 10 days

- Low levels of potassium, phosphate, or magnesium before feeding

Or patient has 2 or more of the following:

- BMI less than 18.5 kg/m^2

- Unintentional weight loss greater than 10% within the previous 3–6 months

- Little or no nutritional intake for more than 5 days

- A history of alcohol abuse or current use of drugs, including insulin, chemotherapy, antacids, or diuretics

Data from National Institute for Health and Clinical Excellence. Nutrition support in adults, in Clinical Guideline. 2006.

monohydrate, CoQ enzyme 10 and vitamin E have been scientifically tested. Approximately 75% of ALS patients are taking dietary supplements[125] based primarily on anecdotal evidence in the hopes of potential efficacy, despite the absence of evidence-based research. **Table 1** groups supplements based on their proposed biologic action. Much of the available research regarding dietary supplements has been completed using ALS animal models, but the few completed clinical trials have not shown benefit. There is no clear evidence that any one supplement or combination of supplements promotes disease reversal or prolongs survival. Additionally, there are few reports of adverse drug-related events occurring from the use of most nutritional supplements, and often the use of these products provides patients with a sense that they are in control of some small aspect of an otherwise uncontrollable process and actively contributing to the management of their disease.

SUMMARY

ALS is a progressive neurodegenerative disease that requires care be provided for ongoing nutrition assessment and management. Malnutrition is a significant comorbidity of ALS, conferring poorer prognosis in this hypermetabolic, physically compromised patient population. The body of literature regarding the significance of adequate nutrition and the consequences of poor nutrition in ALS is growing but comprehensive guidelines for treatment through the progression of the disease are lacking and necessary. Current literature supports the following: malnutrition can be defined as greater than 10% loss of body weight or a BMI less than 20 in certain age groups; if indirect calorimetry is not available to determine a patient's caloric needs, the Harris-Benedict equation provides a reasonable energy requirement estimate by adding an additional 10% to the cREE; RIG placement is likely the safest procedure for providing access for delivery of nutrients and water when swallow is compromised and the nutritional needs of patients are not met by oral intake; and RFS needs to be considered as a potential complication after gastrostomy tube placement in malnourished ALS patients to prevent morbidity and potentially reduce early post–gastrostomy tube placement–associated mortality. Further studies are needed to determine the incidence of RFS in the ALS population and to determine if treatment strategies provide improvement in early post–gastrostomy tube placement associated mortality. There are insufficient data to provide recommendations for the use of dietary supplementation in ALS.

REFERENCES

1. Piquet MA. Nutritional approach for patients with amyotrophic lateral sclerosis. Rev Neurol (Paris) 2006;162(Spec No 2):4S177–4S187 [in French].
2. Jeejeebhoy KN. Muscle function and nutrition. Gut 1986;27(Suppl 1):25–39.
3. Laaban JP, Kouchakji B, Dore MF, et al. Nutritional status of patients with chronic obstructive pulmonary disease and acute respiratory failure. Chest 1993;103(5): 1362–8.
4. Kasarskis EJ, Berryman S, Vanderleest JG, et al. Nutritional status of patients with amyotrophic lateral sclerosis: relation to the proximity of death. Am J Clin Nutr 1996;63(1):130–7.
5. Desport JC, Preux PM, Truong CT, et al. Nutritional assessment and survival in ALS patients. Amyotroph Lateral Scler Other Motor Neuron Disord 2000;1(2): 91–6.

6. Heffernan C, Jenkinson C, Holmes T, et al. Nutritional management in MND/ALS patients: an evidence based review. Amyotroph Lateral Scler Other Motor Neuron Disord 2004;5(2):72–83.
7. Desport JC, Preux PM, Truong TC, et al. Nutritional status is a prognostic factor for survival in ALS patients. Neurology 1999;53(5):1059–63.
8. Heymsfield SB, Tighe A, Wang ZM. Nutritional assessment by anthropometric and biochemical methods. In: Shils ME, Olson JA, Shike M, editors. Modern nutirition in health and disease. Philadelphia: Lea & Febiger; 1994. p. 821–41.
9. Slowie LA, Paige MS, Antel JP. Nutritional considerations in the management of patients with amyotrophic lateral sclerosis (ALS). J Am Diet Assoc 1983;83(1):44–7.
10. Mazzini L, Corra T, Zaccala M, et al. Percutaneous endoscopic gastrostomy and enteral nutrition in amyotrophic lateral sclerosis. J Neurol 1995;242(10):695–8.
11. Marin B, Desport JC, Kajeu P, et al. Alteration of nutritional status at diagnosis is a prognostic factor for survival of amyotrophic lateral sclerosis patients. J Neurol Neurosurg Psychiatry 2011;82(6):628–34.
12. Desport JC, Preux PM, Truong CT, et al. Nutritional status is a prognostic factor for survival in patients with amyotrophic lateral sclerosis. In Proceedings of 9th International Symposium on ALS/MND. Munich (Germany); 1998.
13. Paganoni S, Deng J, Jaffa M, et al. Body mass index, not dyslipidemia, is an independent predictor of survival in amyotrophic lateral sclerosis. Muscle Nerve 2011;44(1):20–4.
14. Frisancho AR. New norms of upper limb fat and muscle areas for assessment of nutritional status. Am J Clin Nutr 1981;34(11):2540–5.
15. Gibson R. Principles of nutritional assessment. New York: Oxford University Press; 1990.
16. Heymsfield SB, McManus C, Stevens V, et al. Muscle mass: reliable indicator of protein-energy malnutrition severity and outcome. Am J Clin Nutr 1982;35(Suppl 5):1192–9.
17. Heymsfield SB, McManus C, Smith J, et al. Anthropometric measurement of muscle mass: revised equations for calculating bone-free arm muscle area. Am J Clin Nutr 1982;36(4):680–90.
18. Kasarskis EJ, Berryman S, English T, et al. The use of upper extremity anthropometrics in the clinical assessment of patients with amyotrophic lateral sclerosis. Muscle Nerve 1997;20(3):330–5.
19. Desport JC, Preux PM, Bouteloup-Demange C, et al. Validation of bioelectrical impedance analysis in patients with amyotrophic lateral sclerosis. Am J Clin Nutr 2003;77(5):1179–85.
20. Kanda F, Fujii Y, Takahashi K, et al. Dual-energy X-ray absorptiometry in neuro-musclular diseases. Muscle Nerve 1994;17:431–5.
21. Nau KL, Bromberg MB, Forshew DA, et al. Individuals with amyotrophic lateral sclerosis are in caloric balance despite losses in mass. J Neurol Sci 1995;129(Suppl):47–9.
22. Tandan R, Krusinki PB, Hiser JR. The validity and sensitivity of dual energy X-ray absorptiometry in estimating lean body mass in amyotrophic lateral sclerosis. In Proceedings of the International Symposium on ALS/MND. Munich (Germany): ALS Association; 1998.
23. Patel BP, Hamadeh MJ. Nutritional and exercise-based interventions in the treatment of amyotrophic lateral sclerosis. Clin Nutr 2009;28(6):604–17.
24. Klein S, Kinney J, Jeejeebhoy K, et al. Nutrition support in clinical practice: review of published data and recommendations for future research directions. National Institutes of Health, American Society for Parenteral and Enteral

Nutrition, and American Society for Clinical Nutrition. JPEN J Parenter Enteral Nutr 1997;21(3):133–56.

25. Jawaid A, Salamone AR, Strutt AM, et al. ALS disease onset may occur later in patients with pre-morbid diabetes mellitus. Eur J Neurol 2010;17(5):733–9.

26. Dupuis L, Corcia P, Fergani A, et al. Dyslipidemia is a protective factor in amyotrophic lateral sclerosis. Neurology 2008;70(13):1004–9.

27. Dorst J, Kuhnlein P, Hendrich C, et al. Patients with elevated triglyceride and cholesterol serum levels have a prolonged survival in amyotrophic lateral sclerosis. J Neurol 2011;258(4):613–7.

28. Sutedja NA, van der Schouw YT, Fischer K, et al. Beneficial vascular risk profile is associated with amyotrophic lateral sclerosis. J Neurol Neurosurg Psychiatry 2011;82(6):638–42.

29. Ikeda K, Hirayama T, Takazawa T, et al. Relationships between disease progression and serum levels of lipid, urate, creatinine and ferritin in Japanese patients with amyotrophic lateral sclerosis: a cross-sectional study. Intern Med 2012; 51(12):1501–8.

30. Chio A, Calvo A, Ilardi A, et al. Lower serum lipid levels are related to respiratory impairment in patients with ALS. Neurology 2009;73(20):1681–5.

31. Kostic Dedic SI, Stevic Z, Dedic V, et al. Is hyperlipidemia correlated with longer survival in patients with amyotrophic lateral sclerosis? Neurol Res 2012;34(6): 576–80.

32. Golomb BA, Kwon EK, Koperski S, et al. Amyotrophic lateral sclerosis-like conditions in possible association with cholesterol-lowering drugs: an analysis of patient reports to the University of California, San Diego (UCSD) Statin Effects Study. Drug Saf 2009;32(8):649–61.

33. Sorensen HT, Lash TL. Statins and amyotrophic lateral sclerosis–the level of evidence for an association. J Intern Med 2009;266(6):520–6.

34. Zinman L, Sadeghi R, Gawel M, et al. Are statin medications safe in patients with ALS? Amyotroph Lateral Scler 2008;9(4):223–8.

35. Glantzounis GK, Tsimoyiannis EC, Kappas AM, et al. Uric acid and oxidative stress. Curr Pharm Des 2005;11(32):4145–51.

36. Scott GS, Cuzzocrea S, Genovese T, et al. Uric acid protects against secondary damage after spinal cord injury. Proc Natl Acad Sci U S A 2005; 102(9):3483–8.

37. Amaro S, Planas AM, Chamorro A. Uric acid administration in patients with acute stroke: a novel approach to neuroprotection. Expert Rev Neurother 2008;8(2):259–70.

38. Paganoni S, Zhang M, Quiroz Zarate A, et al. Uric acid levels predict survival in men with amyotrophic lateral sclerosis. J Neurol 2012. [Epub ahead of print].

39. Lawton KA, Cudkowicz ME, Brown MV, et al. Biochemical alterations associated with ALS. Amyotroph Lateral Scler 2012;13(1):110–8.

40. Ferrannini E. The theoretical bases of indirect calorimetry: a review. Metabolism 1988;37(3):287–301.

41. Mifflin MD, St Jeor ST, Hill LA, et al. A new predictive equation for resting energy expenditure in healthy individuals. Am J Clin Nutr 1990;51(2):241–7.

42. Ellis AC, Rosenfeld J. Which equation best predicts energy expenditure in amyotrophic lateral sclerosis? J Am Diet Assoc 2011;111(11):1680–7.

43. Harris JA, Benedict FG. A biometric study of basal metabolism in man. Proc Natl Acad Sci U S A 1918;4:370–3.

44. Desport JC, Torny F, Lacoste M, et al. Hypermetabolism in ALS: correlations with clinical and paraclinical parameters. Neurodegener Dis 2005;2(3–4):202–7.

45. Bouteloup C, Desport JC, Clavelou P, et al. Hypermetabolism in ALS patients: an early and persistent phenomenon. J Neurol 2009;256(8):1236–42.
46. Sherman MS, Pillai A, Jackson A, et al. Standard equations are not accurate in assessing resting energy expenditure in patients with amyotrophic lateral sclerosis. JPEN J Parenter Enteral Nutr 2004;28(6):442–6.
47. Desport JC, Preux PM, Magy L, et al. Factors correlated with hypermetabolism in patients with amyotrophic lateral sclerosis. Am J Clin Nutr 2001;74(3):328–34.
48. Bosy-Westphal A, Kossel E, Goele K, et al. Contribution of individual organ mass loss to weight loss-associated decline in resting energy expenditure. Am J Clin Nutr 2009; 90(4):993–1001.
49. Weijs PJ. Hypermetabolism, is it real? The example of amyotrophic lateral sclerosis. J Am Diet Assoc 2011;111(11):1670–3.
50. Vaisman N, Lusaus M, Nefussy B, et al. Do patients with amyotrophic lateral sclerosis (ALS) have increased energy needs? J Neurol Sci 2009;279(1–2): 26–9.
51. Funalot B, Desport JC, Sturtz F, et al. High metabolic level in patients with familial amyotrophic lateral sclerosis. Amyotroph Lateral Scler 2009;10(2): 113–7.
52. Shimizu T, Hayashi H, Tanabe H. Energy metabolism of ALS patients under mechanical ventilation and tube feeding. Rinsho Shinkeigaku 1991;31(3): 255–9 [in Japanese].
53. Markus HS, Cox M, Tomkins AM. Raised resting energy expenditure in Parkinson's disease and its relationship to muscle rigidity. Clin Sci (Lond) 1992; 83(2):199–204.
54. Chiang PM, Ling J, Jeong YH, et al. Deletion of TDP-43 down-regulates Tbc1d1, a gene linked to obesity, and alters body fat metabolism. Proc Natl Acad Sci U S A 2010;107(37):16320–4.
55. Xu YF, Gendron TF, Zhang YJ, et al. Wild-type human TDP-43 expression causes TDP-43 phosphorylation, mitochondrial aggregation, motor deficits, and early mortality in transgenic mice. J Neurosci 2010;30(32):10851–9.
56. Shan X, Chiang PM, Price DL, et al. Altered distributions of Gemini of coiled bodies and mitochondria in motor neurons of TDP-43 transgenic mice. Proc Natl Acad Sci U S A 2010;107(37):16325–30.
57. Dupuis L, et al. Up-regulation of mitochondrial uncoupling protein 3 reveals an early muscular metabolic defect in amyotrophic lateral sclerosis. FASEB J 2003; 17(14):2091–3.
58. Gonzalez de Aguilar JL, et al. Gene profiling of skeletal muscle in an amyotrophic lateral sclerosis mouse model. Physiol Genomics 2008;32(2):207–18.
59. Dupuis L, Oudart H, Rene F, et al. Evidence for defective energy homeostasis in amyotrophic lateral sclerosis: benefit of a high-energy diet in a transgenic mouse model. Proc Natl Acad Sci U S A 2004;101(30):11159–64.
60. Echaniz-Laguna A, Zoll J, Ponsot E, et al. Muscular mitochondrial function in amyotrophic lateral sclerosis is progressively altered as the disease develops: a temporal study in man. Exp Neurol 2006;198(1):25–30.
61. Echaniz-Laguna A, Zoll J, Ribera F, et al. Mitochondrial respiratory chain function in skeletal muscle of ALS patients. Ann Neurol 2002;52(5):623–7.
62. Crugnola V, Lamperti C, Lucchini V, et al. Mitochondrial respiratory chain dysfunction in muscle from patients with amyotrophic lateral sclerosis. Arch Neurol 2010;67(7):849–54.
63. Hervias I, Beal MF, Manfredi G. Mitochondrial dysfunction and amyotrophic lateral sclerosis. Muscle Nerve 2006;33(5):598–608.

64. Dobrowolny G, Aucello M, Rizzuto E, et al. Skeletal muscle is a primary target of SOD1G93A-mediated toxicity. Cell Metab 2008;8(5):425–36.

65. Boillee S, Vande Velde C, Cleveland DW. ALS: a disease of motor neurons and their nonneuronal neighbors. Neuron 2006;52(1):39–59.

66. Dupuis L, Pradat PF, Ludolph AC, et al. Energy metabolism in amyotrophic lateral sclerosis. Lancet Neurol 2011;10(1):75–82.

67. Sunderland S, Ray L. Denervation changes in mammalian striated muscle. J Neurol Neurosurg Psychiatry 1959;13:159–77.

68. Csukly K, Ascah A, Matas J, et al. Muscle denervation promotes opening of the permeability transition pore and increases the expression of cyclophilin D. J Physiol 2006;574(Pt 1):319–27.

69. Tews DS. Apoptosis and muscle fibre loss in neuromuscular disorders. Neuromuscul Disord 2002;12(7–8):613–22.

70. Muller FL, Song W, Jang YC, et al. Denervation-induced skeletal muscle atrophy is associated with increased mitochondrial ROS production. Am J Physiol Regul Integr Comp Physiol 2007;293(3):R1159–68.

71. Adhihetty PJ, O'Leary MF, Chabi B, et al. Effect of denervation on mitochondrially mediated apoptosis in skeletal muscle. J Appl Physiol 2007;102(3):1143–51.

72. Joza N, Oudit GY, Brown D, et al. Muscle-specific loss of apoptosis-inducing factor leads to mitochondrial dysfunction, skeletal muscle atrophy, and dilated cardiomyopathy. Mol Cell Biol 2005;25(23):10261–72.

73. Muscaritoli M, Kushta I, Molfino A, et al. Nutritional and metabolic support in patients with amyotrophic lateral sclerosis. Nutrition 2012. [Epub ahead of print].

74. Robbins J. Swallowing in ALS and motor neuron disorders. Neurol Clin 1987;5(2):213–29.

75. Janzen V, Rae R, Hudson A. Otolaryngologic manifestations of amyotrophic lateral sclerosis. J Otolaryngol 1988;17:201–22.

76. Borasio GD, Voltz R. Palliative care in amyotrophic lateral sclerosis. J Neurol 1997;244(Suppl 4):S11–7.

77. Kawai S, Tsukuda M, Mochimatsu I, et al. A study of the early stage of dysphagia in amyotrophic lateral sclerosis. Dysphagia 2003;18(1):1–8.

78. Higo R, Tayama N, Nito T. Longitudinal analysis of progression of dysphagia in amyotrophic lateral sclerosis. Auris Nasus Larynx 2004;31(3):247–54.

79. Traynor BJ, Codd MB, Corr B, et al. Incidence and prevalence of ALS in Ireland, 1995-1997: a population-based study. Neurology 1999;52(3):504–9.

80. Ferguson TA, Elman LB. Clinical presentation and diagnosis of amyotrophic lateral sclerosis. NeuroRehabilitation 2007;22(6):409–16.

81. Langton HR. The management of motor neuron disease in motor neuron disease. In: Leigh PN, Swash M, editors. Biology and management. London: Springer-Verlag; 1995. p. 375–406.

82. Hillel AD, Miller RM. Management of bulbar symptoms in amyotrophic lateral sclerosis. Adv Exp Med Biol 1987;209:201–21.

83. Hardiman O. Symptomatic treatment of respiratory and nutritional failure in amyotrophic lateral sclerosis. J Neurol 2000;247(4):245–51.

84. Leder SB, Novella S, Patwa H. Use of fiberoptic endoscopic evaluation of swallowing (FEES) in patients with amyotrophic lateral sclerosis. Dysphagia 2004;19(3):177–81.

85. Silani V, Kasarskis EJ, Yanagisawa N. Nutritional management in amyotrophic lateral sclerosis: a worldwide perspective. J Neurol 1998;245(Suppl 2):S13–9 [discussion: S29].

86. Mitsumoto H. Nutritional management. In: Mitsumoto H, Chad DA, Pioro EP, editors. Amyotrophic lateral sclerosis. Philadelphia: Davis; 1998. p. 421–36.

87. Gonzalez de Aguilar JL, Dupuis L, Oudart H, et al. The metabolic hypothesis in amyotrophic lateral sclerosis: insights from mutant Cu/Zn-superoxide dismutase mice. Biomed Pharmacother 2005;59(4):190–6.

88. Zhao Z, Lange DJ, Voustianiouk A, et al. A ketogenic diet as a potential novel therapeutic intervention in amyotrophic lateral sclerosis. BMC Neurosci 2006; 7:29.

89. Mattson MP, Cutler RG, Camandola S. Energy intake and amyotrophic lateral sclerosis. Neuromolecular Med 2007;9(1):17–20.

90. Burns BL. Nutritional care in disease of the nervous system. In: Mahan LK, Escott-Stump S, editors. Kruses's food, nutrition and diet therapy. 9th edition. Philadelphia: Saunders; 1996. p. 863–88.

91. Leigh PN, Ray-Chaudhuri K. Motor neuron disease. J Neurol Neurosurg Psychiatry 1994;57(8):886–96.

92. Rio A, Ellis C, Shaw C, et al. Nutritional factors associated with survival following enteral tube feeding in patients with motor neurone disease. J Hum Nutr Diet 2010;23(4):408–15.

93. Leigh NP, Abrahams S, Al-Chalabi A, et al. The management of motor neurone disease. J Neurol Neurosurg Psychiatry 2003;74(Suppl IV):iv31–47.

94. Procaccini NJ, Nemergut EC. Percutaneous endoscopic gastrostomy in the patient with amyotrophic lateral sclerosis: risk vs benefit? In: Parrish CR, editor. Nutrition issues in gastroenterology. 2008. p. 24–34.

95. Miller RG, Rosenberg JA, Gelinas DF, et al. Practice parameter: the care of the patient with amyotrophic lateral sclerosis (An evidence-based review). Muscle Nerve 1999;22(8):1104–18.

96. Langmore SE, Kasarskis EJ, Manca ML, et al. Enteral tube feeding for amyotrophic lateral sclerosis/motor neuron disease. Cochrane Database Syst Rev 2006;(4):CD004030.

97. Thornton FJ, Fotheringham T, Alexander M, et al. Amyotrophic lateral sclerosis: enteral nutrition provision–endoscopic or radiologic gastrostomy? Radiology 2002;224(3):713–7.

98. Desport JC, Mabrouk T, Bouillet P, et al. Complications and survival following radiologically and endoscopically-guided gastrostomy in patients with amyotrophic lateral sclerosis. Amyotroph Lateral Scler Other Motor Neuron Disord 2005; 6(2):88–93.

99. Shaw AS, Ampong MA, Rio A, et al. Survival of patients with ALS following institution of enteral feeding is related to pre-procedure oximetry: a retrospective review of 98 patients in a single centre. Amyotroph Lateral Scler 2006;7(1):16–21.

100. Chio A, Galletti R, Finocchiaro C, et al. Percutaneous radiological gastrostomy: a safe and effective method of nutritional tube placement in advanced ALS. J Neurol Neurosurg Psychiatry 2004;75(4):645–7.

101. Kasarskis EJ, Scarlata D, Hill R, et al. A retrospective study of percutaneous endoscopic gastrostomy in ALS patients during the BDNF and CNTF trials. J Neurol Sci 1999;169(1–2):118–25.

102. Mathus-Vliegen LM, Louwerse LS, Merkus MP, et al. Percutaneous endoscopic gastrostomy in patients with amyotrophic lateral sclerosis and impaired pulmonary function. Gastrointest Endosc 1994;40(4):463–9.

103. Gregory S, Siderowf A, Golaszewski AL, et al. Gastrostomy insertion in ALS patients with low vital capacity: respiratory support and survival. Neurology 2002;58(3):485–7.

104. Spataro R, Ficano L, Piccoli F, et al. Percutaneous endoscopic gastrostomy in amyotrophic lateral sclerosis: effect on survival. J Neurol Sci 2011;304(1–2):44–8.

105. Pena MJ, Ravasco P, Machado M, et al. What is the relevance of percutaneous endoscopic gastrostomy on the survival of patients with amyotrophic lateral sclerosis? Amyotroph Lateral Scler 2012. [Epub ahead of print].

106. Forbes RB, Colville S, Swingler RJ. Frequency, timing and outcome of gastrostomy tubes for amyotrophic lateral sclerosis/motor neurone disease–a record linkage study from the Scottish Motor Neurone Disease Register. J Neurol 2004;251(7):813–7.

107. Chio A, Finocchiaro E, Meineri P, et al. Safety and factors related to survival after percutaneous endoscopic gastrostomy in ALS. ALS Percutaneous Endoscopic Gastrostomy Study Group. Neurology 1999;53(5):1123–5.

108. Mitsumoto H, Davidson M, Moore D, et al. Percutaneous endoscopic gastrostomy (PEG) in patients with ALS and bulbar dysfunction. Amyotroph Lateral Scler Other Motor Neuron Disord 2003;4(3):177–85.

109. Miller RG, Jackson CE, Kasarskis EJ, et al. Practice parameter update: the care of the patient with amyotrophic lateral sclerosis: multidisciplinary care, symptom management, and cognitive/behavioral impairment (an evidence-based review): report of the Quality Standards Subcommittee of the American Academy of Neurology. Neurology 2009;73(15):1227–33.

110. Anderson PM, Abrahams S, Borasio GD, et al. EFNS guidelines on the clinical management of amyotrophic lateral sclerosis. Eur J Neurol 2012;19(3):360–75.

111. Volkert D, Berner YN, Berry E, et al. ESPEN guidelines on enteral nutrition: geriatrics. Clin Nutr 2006;25(2):330–60.

112. Gadek JE, DeMichele SJ, Karlstad MD, et al. Effect of enteral feeding with eicosapentaenoic acid, gamma-linolenic acid, and antioxidants in patients with acute respiratory distress syndrome. Enteral Nutrition in ARDS Study Group. Crit Care Med 1999;27(8):1409–20.

113. Singer P, Theilla M, Fisher H, et al. Benefit of an enteral diet enriched with eicosapentaenoic acid and gamma-linolenic acid in ventilated patients with acute lung injury. Crit Care Med 2006;34(4):1033–8.

114. Pontes-Arruda A, Demichele S, Seth A, et al. The use of an inflammation-modulating diet in patients with acute lung injury or acute respiratory distress syndrome: a meta-analysis of outcome data. JPEN J Parenter Enteral Nutr 2008;32(6):596–605.

115. Pontes-Arruda A, Aragao AM, Albuquerque JD. Effects of enteral feeding with eicosapentaenoic acid, gamma-linolenic acid, and antioxidants in mechanically ventilated patients with severe sepsis and septic shock. Crit Care Med 2006; 34(9):2325–33.

116. Stanga Z, Brunner A, Leuenberger M, et al. Nutrition in clinical practice—the refeeding syndrome: illustrative cases and guidelines for prevention and treatment. Eur J Clin Nutr 2008;62(6):687–94.

117. Mehanna H, Nankivell PC, Moledina J, et al. Refeeding syndrome—awareness, prevention and management. Head Neck Oncol 2009;1:4.

118. National Institute for Health and Clinical Excellence, Nutrition support in adults, in Clinical Guideline. 2006.

119. Boateng AA, Sriram K, Meguid MM, et al. Refeeding syndrome: treatment considerations based on collective analysis of literature case reports. Nutrition 2010;26(2):156–67.

120. Khan LU, Ahmed J, Khan S, et al. Refeeding syndrome: a literature review. Gastroenterol Res Pract 2011;2011.

121. Birmingham CL, Puddicombe D, Hlynsky J. Hypomagnesemia during refeeding in anorexia nervosa. Eat Weight Disord 2004;9(3):236–7.
122. Faintuch J, Soriano FG, Ladeira JP, et al. Refeeding procedures after 43 days of total fasting. Nutrition 2001;17(2):100–4.
123. Lubart E, Leibovitz A, Dror Y, et al. Mortality after nasogastric tube feeding initiation in long-term care elderly with oropharyngeal dysphagia–the contribution of refeeding syndrome. Gerontology 2009;55(4):393–7.
124. Dunn MJ, Walser M. Magnesium depletion in normal man. Metabolism 1966; 15(10):884–95.
125. Bradley WG, Anderson F, Gowda N, et al. Changes in the management of ALS since the publication of the AAN ALS practice parameter 1999. Amyotroph Lateral Scler Other Motor Neuron Disord 2004;5(4):240–4.
126. Cameron A, Rosenfeld J. Nutritional issues and supplements in amyotrophic lateral sclerosis and other neurodegenerative disorders. Curr Opin Clin Nutr Metab Care 2002;5(6):631–43.
127. Rosenfeld J, Ellis A. Nutrition and dietary supplements in motor neuron disease. Phys Med Rehabil Clin N Am 2008;19(3):573–89, x.

Bone Health and Associated Metabolic Complications in Neuromuscular Diseases

Nanette C. Joyce, DO[a],*, Lauren P. Hache, MS, CGC[b],
Paula R. Clemens, MD[c,d]

KEYWORDS

• Neuromuscular disease • Bone density • Vitamin D • Glucocorticoids • Scoliosis

KEY POINTS

• Poor bone health is common in patients with neuromuscular disease and is the cause of significant morbidity, including increased fracture rates and severe scoliosis.

• Bone health depends on a complex interplay of both local and distant mechanisms, including genetic, endocrine, neurologic, and lifestyle factors.

• Osteoporosis in neuromuscular disease may be due to disease-specific pathophysiology, but appears to frequently be complicated by hypovitaminosis D with osteomalacia, as evidenced by incomplete improvements in bone density when serum vitamin D is replete.

• The use of glucocorticoids in Duchenne muscular dystrophy extends independent ambulation; however, its effects on bone health have not been completely studied, and may have adverse effects on bone density and increase fracture risk. Further studies are warranted.

• Further research is needed to assess the extent of poor bone health across all neuromuscular disease and to evaluate the efficacy of known osteoporosis treatments in this unique patient population.

The authors take full responsibility for the contents of this article, which do not represent the views of the Department of Veterans Affairs or the United States Government.
Dr Joyce is supported by the Association of Academic Physiatrists and the National Institutes of Health.
[a] Department of Rehabilitation Medicine, University of California, Davis 4860 Y Street, Suite 3850, Sacramento, CA 95817, USA; [b] Center for Genetic Medicine, Children's National Medical Center, 111 Michigan Avenue, Northwest, Washington, DC 20010, USA; [c] Department of Neurology, University of Pittsburgh, S-520 Biomedical Science Tower Pittsburgh, PA 15213, USA; [d] Neurology Service, Department of Veterans Affairs Medical Center, Pittsburgh, PA 15240, USA
* Corresponding author.
E-mail address: Nanette.joyce@ucdmc.ucdavis.edu

Phys Med Rehabil Clin N Am 23 (2012) 773–799
http://dx.doi.org/10.1016/j.pmr.2012.08.005
1047-9651/12/$ – see front matter © 2012 Elsevier Inc. All rights reserved.

pmr.theclinics.com

INTRODUCTION

The Bone and Joint Decade, an international collaborative movement sanctioned by the United Nations and World Health Organization, has focused worldwide attention on the growing burden of musculoskeletal and bone disease.[1] In the United States alone, it is estimated that more than 1 in 4 people will require treatment for a musculoskeletal disorder. Jacobs and colleagues[2] reported that during 2004, the United States spent $849 billion in direct and indirect costs toward bone and joint health, equaling 7.7% of the gross domestic product. As a direct consequence of highlighting this growing public health concern, the Bone and Joint Initiative has increased research focused on unraveling the basic biological mechanisms involved in bone development and maintenance of bone health. Although the literature regarding musculoskeletal and bone disorders in neuromuscular disease (NMD) remains scant, the research advances generated as a result of this movement are relevant to and provide insight for therapeutic approaches. Poor bone health is often a significant problem for patients with NMD.[3] Deficiency of bone mineral density (BMD) and increased incidence of bone fractures, for example, are a well-recognized clinical consequence of diseases such as Duchenne muscular dystrophy (DMD), amyotrophic lateral sclerosis (ALS), and spinal muscular atrophy (SMA).[3–5] A long bone fracture in a patient with NMD often heralds loss of independent ambulation. Furthermore, therapy with corticosteroids, a recommended treatment for DMD, may have deleterious effects on bone health, which has not been extensively explored. The aim of this review is to present the current literature on bone development and health as it relates to the patient diagnosed with an NMD, and to demonstrate the need for disease-specific research to develop both diagnostic and therapeutic treatment strategies aimed at improving bone health and reducing associated morbidity in this population at risk.

NORMAL BONE GROWTH AND DEVELOPMENT
Bone Components and Formation

The skeleton is a dynamic, metabolically active organ that is in constant flux. Our bones serve 2 main functions: a metabolic function, as the reservoir for calcium and phosphate needed for serum homeostasis; and a structural function, housing and protecting vital organs and serving as a strut for muscle attachment, which permits locomotion.[6,7] There are 2 types of bone in the normal, mature human skeleton: cortical and trabecular.[8] Although macroscopically and microscopically different, the 2 forms are identical in their chemical composition.[6] Cortical bone is dense and compact, has a slow turnover rate with high resistance to bending and torsion, and constitutes the outer layer of the bony structure. Trabecular bone is less dense, more elastic, contributes to mechanical support particularly in bones such as the vertebrae, and provides the initial supply of minerals in acute deficiency states. In osteoporosis, a disease characterized by reduced bone strength and increased susceptibility to fractures, trabecular bone is often more severely affected than cortical bone.

The structural components of bone consist of a largely mineralized extracellular matrix, constructed of type I collagen fibers and noncollagenous proteins. The matrix accounts for approximately 90% of the organic composition of the skeleton.[9] The most abundant noncollagenous matrix protein is osteocalcin. Osteocalcin participates in the stabilization of the hydroxyapatite matrix and binds calcium.[9] It is a negative regulator of bone formation and inhibits premature or inappropriate mineralization.[10] By contrast, biglycan, another noncollagenous bone matrix protein, positively regulates bone formation.[11]

Bone Growth

Total skeletal calcium increases from approximately 25 g at birth to 1200 g in early adulthood.[12] These gains are achieved through bone modeling, the process that alters bone length, diameter, and shape during growth. The cells responsible for osteogenesis (the embryonic or postfracture process of bone formation), bone modeling, and bone remodeling are the osteoblast, osteocyte, and osteoclast. Osteoblasts are small, single-nucleated cells that lay new bone distant from the resorption site and line all bone surfaces as "lining cells." As osteoblasts encapsulate themselves in bone matrix during modeling and remodeling, they become quiescent and are then considered osteocytes. Osteoclasts are large multinucleated cells that resorb old or damaged bone beneath the periosteum by acidification and proteolysis of the bone matrix and hydroxyapatite crystals.

Most of the accrual in bone mineral content during growth is due to increases in bone size, rather than density. However, in contrast to cortical bone density, which remains constant across age, gender, and race, trabecular bone increases in density during puberty. The increases in trabecular bone density have been observed in the lumbar spine.[13] Once growth ceases, aged bone is continuously replaced through the process of remodeling, which serves to repair microdamage and maintain skeletal integrity without altering bone size or shape.

Bone Remodeling

Bone remodeling is accomplished by groups of osteoblasts and osteoclasts acting together in concert. This functional group is referred to as the basic multicellular unit.[14] The process of remodeling is thought to be activated by osteoblast lineage cells including the lining cells, mesenchymal stem cells located within bone marrow, and osteocytes. Evidence suggests that osteocytes are the primary mediator of the remodeling cycle.[15] However, each of these cells secrete receptor activator nuclear factor κB ligand (RANKL), a protein belonging to the tumor necrosis factor (TNF) superfamily, which initiates fusion of osteoclast lineage cells producing mature osteoclasts.[16] Osteoclast precursor cell fusion occurs through the interaction of RANKL and RANK, an osteocyte lineage cell surface binding site.[17] The processes leading to cell fusion are inhibited by both osteoprotegerin (OPG), a dimeric glycoprotein that functions as a decoy receptor and blocks the RANKL-RANK interaction, and sclerostin, a glycoprotein antagonist of the Wnt signaling pathway. OPG and sclerostin are mainly produced and secreted by osteoblast lineage cells.[15,18,19] The OPG-RANKL-RANK interactions illustrate mechanisms of local control and coupling of bone formation and resorption cycles.

In children, bone formation typically outpaces resorption, whereas in the young adult bone formation is coupled to resorption. With aging and in many pathologic bone conditions, resorption shifts to exceed formation, resulting in a negative bone balance and loss of BMD.

Growth, development, and maintenance of healthy bone are controlled by a complex multifactorial process with both local and distant regulation including genetic, endocrine, neurologic, and lifestyle influences. Disturbances in any component of this well-integrated process may cause marked alterations in bone modeling and remodeling, often resulting in abnormal bone density and increased risk of fracture.

DETERMINANTS OF BONE MASS

A brief overview of selected aspects of the physiologic processes involved in bone acquisition and maintenance of bone density is presented here. Many of these processes are likely to be disturbed in patients with NMD and may suggest some rationales for treatments aimed at improving bone health.

Genetic Factors

Numerous factors are important in influencing the achievement of maximum bone height and density. However, bone size potential for an individual, as defined as the size a bone can reach under optimal circumstances, is determined by genetic factors. There have been considerable advances made over the past decade toward understanding the genetic basis of bone development and maintenance. However, the scope of this review encompasses the introduction of a signaling pathway necessary for normal bone metabolism. The interested reader is encouraged to read the review by Karsenty and colleagues,[20] which covers the topic in greater depth.

Wnts are an evolutionarily conserved family of growth factors whose signaling is involved in numerous processes, including bone formation and maintenance.[21] The Wnt/β-catenin pathway plays a crucial role in bone formation and generally promotes an increase in bone mass by mechanisms including renewal of stem cells, osteoblast proliferation, induction of osteoblast formation, and inhibition of osteoblast and osteocyte apoptosis.[22]

Endocrine Factors

Parathyroid hormone

Parathyroid hormone (PTH) is released from chief cells in the parathyroid glands when the plasma calcium concentration decreases, acting as the key regulator of calcium and phosphate homeostasis. The direct actions of PTH on kidney and bone, or the indirect actions on the intestines contribute to restoring the concentration of plasma calcium.[23] These responses are mediated by parathyroid receptors that bind PTH.[24] The response of bone depends on interactions between osteoblasts and osteoclasts, as only osteoblasts express the parathyroid receptor, and is variable depending on PTH secretion patterns.[25] In experimental models of osteoporosis in which bone loss was induced by ovariectomy, intermittent treatment with PTH led to increased osteoblastic activity, with recovery of bone density.[26,27] When secreted continuously, however, PTH induced osteoblast-osteoclast coupling factors, promoting resorption by increasing secretion of RANKL.[28]

PTH is the first anabolic drug to be approved for the treatment of osteoporosis. Tu and colleagues[29] recently reported results from a small prospective trial in which patients with a history of multiple osteoporotic vertebral compression fractures were followed. None of the 28 patients treated with PTH, over a period of at least 18 months, experienced new-onset vertebral fracture, and vertebral bone density increased.

Calcitonin

Calcitonin is produced by the parafollicular C cells of the thyroid gland. High levels of plasma calcium stimulate secretion of calcitonin, which activates renal calcium excretion and impairs osteoclast function. The downstream effects, mediated by calcitonin receptors found on osteoclasts, promote bone formation by reducing osteoclast motility, bone-surface binding, and proteolytic enzyme secretion.[30] Calcitonin nasal spray has demonstrated the ability to decrease fracture risk and has been approved by the Food and Drug Administration for the treatment of osteoporosis since 1995. Oral preparations have been in development; however, after an initial successful 3-month phase 2 multicenter, randomized, double-blind, placebo-controlled dose-ranging trial demonstrating reduced serum and urine bone turnover markers

(BTMs), Novartis announced in late 2011 that their 3-year phase 3 multicenter trial did not produce significant reductions in vertebral or nonvertebral fracture risk.[31]

Androgen hormones

Androgen hormones are necessary for normal growth and maintenance of bone health. Androgen receptors are ubiquitously expressed across bone cell types.[32,33] The role that androgens play in bone modeling has been well explored in animal and human studies over the last 3 decades. Testosterone increases skeletal calcium uptake in prepubertal boys, and testosterone therapy has been shown in both prospective and retrospective studies of male hypogonadism to increase bone density.[34,35] Androgens influence longitudinal bone growth during early puberty and epiphyseal growth-plate closure in later puberty by direct effects on growth-plate chondrocytes. Under strict culture conditions, Carrascosa and colleagues[36] demonstrated that androgens regulate both proliferation and differentiation of cultured epiphyseal chondrocytes. In addition, androgens appear to have indirect effects on pituitary function, shifting the kinetics of growth-hormone secretion during puberty.[37]

Estrogen hormones

Estrogen receptors are expressed within the human growth plate. Studies have confirmed that epiphyseal closure during late puberty depends on estrogen in both males and females.[38–42] Estrogens appear to play a greater role than testosterone in preventing bone loss in elderly men, and testosterone's effects may be indirect and mediated through the estrogen receptor, as testosterone is metabolized via the cytochrome P450 aromatase enzyme complex into 17β-estradiol.[43,44] In one uncontrolled study of eugonadal men, Anderson and colleagues[45] showed that testosterone therapy appeared to exert its beneficial effects mainly through increased levels of serum estrogen, as estrogen levels increased more than serum testosterone levels.

Estrogen decreases the responsiveness of osteoclast progenitor cells to RANKL, preventing osteoclast formation and shortening the life span of osteoclasts. Estrogen affects genes coding for enzymes, bone-matrix proteins, hormone receptors, and transcription factors. Estrogen also upregulates the production of OPG, insulin-like growth factors, and tissue growth factor β, promoting bone formation.[46]

Glucocorticoids

The role of glucocorticoids in bone health and disease is complex, with both stimulatory and inhibitory effects on bone cells.[6] Glucocorticoids are important for the normal regulation of bone remodeling and are essential for osteoblast differentiation from mesenchymal stem cells. Glucocorticoids influence osteoblast gene expression, including downregulation of type I collagen and osteocalcin, and upregulation of interstitial collagenase. The synthesis of osteoblast growth factors are modulated by glucocorticoids. For example, the expression of insulin-like growth factor I, an important osteoblast trophic factor, is decreased by glucocorticoids.[47]

Glucocorticoids can have varying and quite opposing effects on bone.[48] Whereas endogenous glucocorticoids at appropriate physiologic levels are necessary for normal bone health and development, abnormally increased endogenous secretion or pharmacologic glucocorticoids induce bone loss and promote osteoporosis.[49,50] Prolonged exposure to excess glucocorticoids is the most common cause of secondary osteoporosis.[51] Clinically, patients with glucocorticoid-induced osteoporosis develop bone loss within the first few months of glucocorticoid exposure.[52] It has been reported that bone loss occurs with a rapid phase of about 12% within the first year of glucocorticoid administration, followed by a slow phase of 2% to 5% annually.[53–55] Multiple practice guidelines have been written recommending treatment protocols for patients, including those diagnosed with DMD who are placed on chronic glucocorticoid treatment, to reduce fractures and the morbidity associated with glucocorticoid-induced osteoporosis (**Tables 1** and **2**).[56,57]

Thyroid hormones

Thyroid hormones are required for skeletal development and the establishment of peak bone mass. Population studies indicate that both hypothyroidism and hyperthyroidism are associated with increased fracture risk.[58] Growth retardation and delayed skeletal development occur in children who are hypothyroid. Hyperthyroidism increases renal excretion of calcium and phosphorus, resulting in bone loss. Therefore, maintaining a euthyroid state is essential for bone health.[59,60] The processes by which thyroid hormone alters bone metabolism are not fully understood; however, increasing evidence exists to suggest a dependent interplay between thyroid hormone, insulin-like growth factor I, and the Wtn/β-catenin signaling pathway.[61]

Neurologic Factors

Neurons and neurotransmitters are intimately involved in bone remodeling. Bones have abundant innervation with nerve processes running along vessels adjacent to bone trabeculae, where terminal nerve boutons are in contact with bone cells.[62] Discovery of β2 adrenergic receptors and receptors for neurotransmitters such as glutamate and Neuromedin U, on both osteoblasts and osteoclasts, suggests a critical homeostatic role of the peripheral nervous system in the regulation of bone metabolism.[63,64] In addition, central nervous system influence on bone metabolism has been linked to the hypothalamus through a Leptin-β2 adrenergic receptor–dependent system. Leptin is a 16-kDa peptide hormone synthesized by adipocytes, which affects appetite and energy metabolism through its binding to the leptin receptor located in the hypothalamus.[65,66] Mice lacking a functional Leptin receptor are obese and sterile,

Table 1
Recommendations for monitoring patients receiving glucocorticoid therapy for a duration of 3 months or longer

Screening Categories	American College of Rheumatology	DMD Care Consideration
Bone density	Consider serial BMD testing	Annual BMD testing
Serum 25-hydroxyvitamin D	Consider annual serum 25-hydroxyvitamin D screening	Annual 25-hydroxyvitamin D screening in late winter
Height	Annual height measurement	Height screening every 6 mo
Fracture	Assessment of incident fragility fracture	Take a careful fracture history
Medication compliance	Assessment of osteoporosis medication compliance	No recommendation
Glucocorticoid treatment side effects	No recommendation	Screen for additional side effects with regular follow-up

Data from Grossman JM, Gordon R, Ranganath VK, et al. American College of Rheumatology 2010 recommendations for the prevention and treatment of glucocorticoid-induced osteoporosis. Arthritis Care Res (Hoboken) 2010;62(11):1515–26; and Bushby K, Finkel R, Birnkrant DJ, et al. Diagnosis and management of Duchenne muscular dystrophy, part 1: diagnosis, and pharmacological and psychosocial management. Lancet Neurol 2010;9(1):77–93.

Table 2
Recommendations for adjunctive treatment of patients receiving glucocorticoid therapy

Treatment Category	American College of Rheumatology	DMD Care Considerations
Vitamin D	Supplement vitamin D	Supplement with vitamin D_3 if serum level is less than 32 nmol/L: If between 20 and 31 nmol/L give 1000 IU orally twice daily If less than 20 nmol/L give 2000 IU orally twice daily Recheck serum 25-hydroxyvitamin D after 3 mo of treatment
Calcium	Calcium intake 1200–1500 mg/d	No recommendation
Physical activity	Encourage weight-bearing activities	Encourage weight-bearing activities
Lifestyle modification	Avoid: tobacco, alcohol >2 drinks per day	No recommendation
Osteoporosis medications	If glucocorticoid dose 7.5 mg/d or more and treatment will be at least 3 mo: add alendronate, risedronate, or zoledronic acid If high fracture risk, may treat with teriparatide	Consider treatment with a bisphosphonate, such as pamidronate

Data from Grossman JM, Gordon R, Ranganath VK, et al. American College of Rheumatology 2010 recommendations for the prevention and treatment of glucocorticoid-induced osteoporosis. Arthritis Care Res (Hoboken) 2010;62(11):1515–26; and Bushby K, Finkel R, Birnkrant DJ, et al. Diagnosis and management of Duchenne muscular dystrophy, part 1: diagnosis, and pharmacological and psychosocial management. Lancet Neurol 2010;9(1):77–93.

and despite hypogonadism, the most common cause of osteoporosis, have high bone mass.[67] The central signals mediated by Leptin are relayed through the sympathetic nervous system and target osteoblasts expressing β2 adrenergic receptors. In support of these findings, mice treated with isoproterenol, a β agonist, displayed a massive decrease in bone mass. Conversely, mice with blocked sympathetic nervous system signaling had high bone mass.[68,69] β2 Adrenergic receptors also control osteoblast expression of both RANKL and mRNA for factors that promote bone resorption.[70]

Ma and colleagues[71] recently demonstrated that dexamethasone, a glucocorticoid, stimulates the expression of β2 adrenergic receptors in differentiated primary calvarial osteoblasts after short-term treatment. In addition, their results confirmed both an accumulation of isoproterenol-induced cyclic adenosine monophosphate and increased expression of RANKL. The dexamethasone treatment appeared to promote the general responsiveness of the osteoblasts to adrenergic stimulation, suggesting that glucocorticoid-induced bone loss may be mediated by alterations in the tonic state of sympathetic signal receptivity, favoring bone resorption.

Lifestyle Factors

Nutrition

Calcium and vitamin D Calcium and vitamin D play a critical role in skeletal development and continuing bone health. Calcium is required for the maintenance of bone health. The amount of calcium required to meet the needs of the body changes throughout childhood and into adulthood, with peak nutritional needs occurring during adolescence.[72] During periods of slower growth, the relationship between urinary calcium excretion and calcium intake is more pronounced than during the period of rapid growth in adolescence when calcium need is high.

Vitamin D nutrition Vitamin D is essential for facilitating calcium absorption.[73] Calcium regulation and the 25-hydroxyvitamin D–PTH axis is well established, and is illustrated by the inverse relationship between serum 25-hydroxyvitamin D and serum PTH. Severe vitamin D deficiency causes rickets or osteomalacia whereby new bone is poorly mineralized, causing bone softening and deformity. Less severe vitamin D deficiency often results in increased serum PTH leading to bone resorption, osteoporosis, and increased risk of fracture.[74] The NHANES study compared the risk of hip fractures in adults for several ranges of serum 25-hydroxyvitamin D levels: below 16 ng/mL, risk of hip fracture was 60% higher; between 16 and 20 ng/mL it was 45% higher; between 20 and 25 ng/mL fracture risk was 36% higher; and between 25 and 30 ng/mL there was a nonsignificant increased risk of hip fracture of 13%.[75] Two meta-analyses, published within the past 5 years, evaluated the effect of both vitamin D and calcium supplementation on bone health and fracture risk. These studies included a total of 114,625 adults from vitamin D–insufficient regions. The analyses concluded that vitamin D alone was not effective in reducing fracture rate (hazard ratio, 1.01; 95% confidence interval, 0.92–1.12); however, vitamin D intake of at least 800 IU/d combined with a calcium intake of 1000 to 1200 mg/d was effective for fracture prevention.[76,77]

Sources of vitamin D include direct skin exposure to sunlight, few foods, and dietary supplements. Skin exposure to ultraviolet B radiation from the sun provides the predominant source of vitamin D. An individual in a bathing suit generates 10,000 to 25,000 IU of vitamin D2 after 1 minimal erythemal dose, which is the safest amount of radiation sufficient to produce redness in the skin.[78] After hydroxylation in the liver and kidney to 25-hydroxyvitamin D and 1,25-dihydroxyvitamin D, respectively, the active metabolite binds to the vitamin D receptor in a cell, and induces transcription of a responsive gene. Calcium-binding protein is a product of vitamin D–induced transcription, and mediates calcium transport across the intestinal mucosa.

The vitamin D receptor has been found in many tissues including bone and muscle cells, suggesting wide physiologic influence. The half-life of 25-hydroxyvitamin D in the body is approximately 15 to 20 days.[79] In 2011, the Institute of Medicine (IOM) published recommendations, derived from a thorough review of the current literature, for the daily intake of vitamin D and calcium for children and adults. The IOM increased the 2008 American Academy of Pediatrics recommendations for vitamin D from 400 IU/d to 600 IU/d for children and adults 1 to 70 years old, and 800 IU/d for seniors older than 70 years.[80] In a prospective trial assessing treatment response, 400 IU/d of vitamin D increased the serum 25-hydroxyvitamin D level in postmenopausal women by an average of 32.5 nmol/L over a 12-month treatment period. This increase was higher than previous predictions suggesting 400 IU/d would only raise serum 25-hydroxyvitamin D by approximately 10 nmol/L.[81] With standard-dose supplementation, serum 25-hydroxyvitamin D is likely to plateau after 3 to 4 months.[82] Therefore, when monitoring a patient's response to supplementation, a serum 25-hydroxyvitamin D should be measured no sooner than 3 months after treatment begins.[83]

The serum concentration of 25-hydroxyvitamin D_3 is considered the best available biomarker to measure the nutritional status of vitamin D. There are multiple assays in use, and clinicians should be aware that studies comparing interassay and interlaboratory testing of serum concentrations of 25-hydroxyvitamin D_3 have revealed significant variability in the results, making the assessment of vitamin D status in patients and the interpretation of vitamin D efficacy studies inherently more difficult.[84–86]

Vitamin K In addition, there is evidence in human intervention studies that vitamins D and K work synergistically toward improving bone density. Vitamin K is required for the γ-carboxylation of osteocalcin.[87] In a recently published study evaluating the combined use of supplemental calcium, vitamin D, and Vitamin K on bone health, greater increases were observed in bone density within the lumbar spine of treated subjects when compared with the control group, who were treated with calcium and vitamin D.[88]

Magnesium Magnesium is the second most abundant intracellular cation, playing an important role in enzyme function and transmembrane ion transport. Magnesium deficiency has been associated with osteoporosis. Rates of magnesium deprivation sufficient to induce osteoporosis in animal studies are thought to occur commonly in the Western diet.[89] Magnesium deficiency has been shown to increase substance P, TNF-α, IL-1β, and RANKL, with a decrease in OPG, favoring increased bone resorption.

Researchers have begun to evaluate multinutrient therapies for the treatment of osteoporosis. Genuis and Bouchard[90] recently published findings from a series of patients who had failed bisphosphonate therapy and were treated using a combination of micronutrients chosen from the literature for their bone health properties. The treatment included 12-month supplementation with vitamin D_3, vitamin K, strontium, magnesium, and docosahexaenoic acid. Serial bone densitometry was performed and demonstrated improved BMD in compliant patients. It was concluded that the supplementation regimen appeared to be at least as effective as bisphosphonates in raising BMD levels in the hip, spine, and femoral neck. No fractures occurred during follow-up in the micronutrient treatment group.

Physical activity

Weight-bearing physical activity is considered an intervention strategy for promoting optimal bone density in youth and to reduce bone loss in adults.[91,92] Dynamic loading promotes greater bone-tissue gains than static loading, even if static loads produce large forces.[93] Athletes involved in high-impact sports such as gymnastics show greater bone density than those involved in low-impact sports such as swimming.[94] Health problems that reduce bone stimulation from mechanical loading result in bone loss, as illustrated by disuse osteoporosis caused by prolonged bed rest and immobilization. Reduction of mechanical stress on bone inhibits osteoblast-mediated bone formation and accelerates osteoclast-mediated bone resorption.[95] Rittweger and colleagues[96] performed a 35-day bed-rest investigation and assessed BMD 2 weeks after the initiation of bed rest, and reported reduction of bone mass in the cancellous bone–rich areas of 1% at the distal femur, 3% at the patella, and 2% at the distal tibia, with no changes seen at the distal radius. Results of a cross-sectional study completed by Garland and colleagues[97] demonstrated more than 20% bone loss at the distal femur 3 months after injury in posttraumatic paraplegic and quadriplegic patients with spinal cord injuries. It is intriguing that high-frequency, low-intensity whole-body vibration has demonstrated bone-improving effects similar to those of mechanical force on bone density in both animal and human studies.[98,99]

FRACTURE RISK ASSESSMENT

Bone quality may be evaluated in several different ways. Dual-energy x-ray absorptiometry (DXA), quantitative computed tomography (QTC), and bone turnover markers

(BTMs) are some examples. QTC is a 3-dimensional nonprojectional technique used to quantify BMD in the spine, proximal femur, forearm, and tibia. There are several advantages of QTC in comparison with other densitometric techniques: cortical and trabecular bone can be separated, trabecular volumes of interest are largely independent of degenerative changes in the spine, and 3-dimensional geometric parameters can be determined.[100] BMD, as measured by QTC, is a true density, measured in g/cm^3, in contrast to DXA, which determines an areal density measured in g/cm^2. However, QTC has not become the standard measure in the clinical setting, where DXA scanning remains the technique of choice for the assessment of pathologic bone conditions. DXA provides reference data from infancy to postpuberty, taking into account effects of age, sex, race, maturation, and size on BMD and bone mineral content (BMC), and allows a determination of the degree of departure from normative values in the form of t- and z-scores. BMD is the standard for evaluating fracture risk and is easily measured in patients. However, DXA provides only an estimate of BMC, and derives the BMD by dividing the BMC by the projected area of bone evaluated. The derived BMD is not a measure of volumetric density, providing no information about the depth of bone. In addition, bones of larger width and height also tend to be thicker, and bone thickness is not factored into DXA estimates of BMD, resulting in underestimates for short individuals.[101] Children, particularly those with smaller bones, may appear to have a mineralization disorder. This effect is clearly important when assessing children's bone health with DXA. In 2011, revised pediatric DXA reference curves were published by Zemel and colleagues[102] derived from their data on 2014 healthy children. These investigators recommended adjusting for height in children, particularly those whose height is at the extremes of the normal growth continuum, and included parameters and an equation to adjust for these differences. However, the revised reference curves have yet to be evaluated as a predictor of fracture risk. Previously reported studies have shown a weak inverse relationship between BMD as determined by DXA and subsequent fracture risk.[103]

MEASURES OF BONE TURNOVER

BTMs are readily detectable peptides released from the bone matrix and through collagen degradation; however, their variability is of practical concern. The release of these substances may reflect bone turnover and indicate abnormalities in bone and mineral metabolism; however, marker concentration does not necessarily correlate with the severity of the mineralization process. Commonly used biomarkers of bone turnover include serum osteocalcin, amino-terminal propeptide of type I procollagen, and urine and serum β-isomerized C-telopeptides.[104] Newer BTMs include P1NP and TRACP5b. P1NP is a marker of early osteoblast proliferation, and TRACP5b is a marker of osteoclastic activity and bone resorption. It is the only form of TRACP enzyme secreted by osteoclasts.

BONE HEALTH IN SELECTED NEUROMUSCULAR DISEASES
Duchenne Muscular Dystrophy

Bone health has been studied more extensively in DMD than in any other NMD, and reports date back to 1941.[105–107] DMD is an X-linked recessive disorder characterized by progressive muscle weakness, leading to premature death. DMD affects about 1 in 3600 to 6000 males and is the most common form of muscular dystrophy.[108,109] The DMD phenotype is caused by a mutation in the dystrophin gene, resulting in the translation of a defective dystrophin protein that is rapidly degraded. This process results in a severe reduction or absence of dystrophin protein within muscle and destabilizing effects on the sarcolemmal membrane.[110]

DMD is typically first recognized in affected boys by 5 years of age. Early signs include calf pseudohypertrophy and proximal leg weakness, which impairs mobility and results in the classic Gower maneuver observed when an affected boy transfers from the floor to standing. By definition, boys diagnosed with a DMD phenotype lose independent ambulation before age 16 years, with the most typical time for transition to wheelchair occurring before the earlier teens. DMD is a multisystem disorder including progressive respiratory and cardiac dysfunction, which are often the sequelae responsible for reduced life expectancy.[57,111]

Decreased BMD and fractures occur commonly in DMD, and have been reported repeatedly.[5,106,107,112–125] The recent shift in consensus recommendations to support routine use of corticosteroids for disease-modifying treatment, aimed at prolonging ambulation in DMD patients, has heightened concern for bone health because of the known negative impact of chronic glucocorticoid treatment in other patient populations. No rigorous studies have been published examining the effects of corticosteroids on bone health in DMD; however, since 2004 a growing number of international workshops have convened to address this issue.[126–130]

Limitations in the current literature addressing bone health in DMD include lack of concurrent age- and sex-matched healthy controls, and variations in study design including methods and outcome measures, which make it difficult to reliably interpret the results reported for many of the biochemical indicators of bone health.

Scoliosis in DMD

Scoliosis has been reported to occur in up to 90% of patients with DMD. It is one of the most obvious observations that dystrophin deficiency has accompanying effects on bone health and development.[131] However, a retrospective study of 143 patients diagnosed with DMD and comparing steroid-treated with steroid-naïve boys revealed an increase in the mean age at transition to wheelchair by approximately 3 years and reduced scoliosis severity, limiting the need for surgical stabilization in the treated group. The mean degree of scoliosis measured in the nontreated group was $33.15° \pm 29.98°$ versus $11.58° \pm 15.65°$ for the treated group ($P<.0001$).[132]

Fractures in DMD

Estimates suggest that up to 25% of boys with DMD will experience a long bone fracture with subsequent loss of ambulation.[118] In a large retrospective study that examined the case reports of 378 boys with DMD, 20.9% or 79 patients had experienced fractures. Falls were the most commonly reported cause of fracture. Of patients with fractures, 48% were between 8 and 11 years old, and 48% were ambulatory. In boys ambulating with the assistance of knee-ankle-foot orthoses, upper limb fractures occurred most commonly (65%). Lower limb fractures were most prevalent in independently mobile and wheelchair-dependent patients (54% and 68%, respectively). Of independently ambulant patients and those using orthoses, 20% and 27%, respectively, lost mobility permanently as a result of the fracture. The investigators reported the fracture prevalence of those exposed to corticosteroids as similar to that of the unexposed group. However, they did not examine steroid regimens or ascertain the interval between corticosteroid initiation and fracture in the study population.[118]

Before the broad initiation of corticosteroid treatment in DMD, reports of vertebral fractures were relatively rare.[117,118] However, recent retrospective studies have reported increased vertebral fracture rates in patients treated with corticosteroids in comparison with steroid-naïve patients (**Fig. 1**).[132] Of the 143 patients studied by King and colleagues,[132] 75 patients had received steroid treatment of at least 1 year's duration, and 68 were steroid naïve. No vertebral fractures were identified in the nontreated group, but 32% of the treated group suffered a vertebral fracture. Another study of 79 DMD patients by Houde and colleagues,[133] including 37 patients treated with deflazacort, reported similar frequencies of limb fractures between deflazacort-treated (24%) and untreated (26%) boys. Vertebral fractures, however, occurred exclusively in the treated group (7 of 37 patients).

In a study of 25 DMD patients who were treated with daily corticosteroids for a median duration of 4.5 years, 40% sustained vertebral fractures. Eight were identified due to symptomatic backache, and 2 had fractures detected on spinal radiographs taken because of low BMD. The first reported fracture occurred at 40 months into treatment.[119] These reports highlight the importance of including fracture surveillance as part of regular follow-up care for the steroid-treated DMD population (see **Table 1**).

BMD in DMD

Many DMD studies have reported decreases in BMD.[114,116,120–123,134] Aparicio and colleagues[116] evaluated the BMD of 10 DMD boys by DXA. None of the boys had been treated with corticosteroids and all were community ambulators between the ages of 6 and 11 years. Eight of the 10 boys had osteoporosis of the proximal femur, and the remaining 2 had abnormal measures more consistent with osteopenia. Two of the 10 patients had decreased BMD of the spine within the osteoporotic range, and 3 were osteopenic. The study did not include aged-matched controls for comparison. In a prospective study where 30 steroid-naïve DMD boys underwent from 2 to 17 DXA evaluations over a 7-year period, Larson and Henderson[114] evaluated BMD through

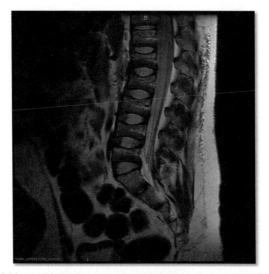

Fig. 1. A 9-year-old boy with DMD treated with chronic glucocorticoids, who has scoliosis and a 3-week history of intermittent lower back pain. Magnetic resonance image of his lumbar spine reveals multilevel vertebral loss of body height with increased prominence of the disc spaces with respect to the vertebral bodies. There is increased T2 signal at the superior endplate of L5 and L1, as well as diffusely in the L2 vertebral body, suggesting marrow edema and more recent fracture.

the time spanning independent ambulation to wheelchair dependence. While ambulatory, the BMD in the lumbar spine was only slightly decreased (mean z-score, −0.8); however, significant decreases occurred in BMD with loss of ambulation (mean z-score, −1.7). By contrast, BMD of the proximal femur was diminished before the loss of ambulation (mean z-score, −1.6), and progressively worsened to nearly 4 standard deviations below age-matched nondiseased controls (mean z-score, −3.9). A study by Söderpalm and colleagues[135] assessed the bone health of 24 boys treated with glucocorticoids in comparison with controls. BMD differed significantly from controls at all ages, and these differences in values between patients and controls increased significantly with age. While the above studies confirm baseline BMD abnormalities in both nonsteroid and steroid-treated DMD patients, the question still remains: do corticosteroids improve baseline BMD by improving muscle strength and prolonging ambulation, or do they have additive bone-deteriorating effects worsening the bone health of DMD boys?

The recent study by Rufo and colleagues,[136] aimed at exploring the mechanism responsible for the deterioration of bone health in DMD, is one of the most comprehensive studies of bone health in DMD to date. The study design incorporated multiple outcome measurements across human subjects, the *mdx* mouse model, and in vitro culture of osteoclast precursors and primary osteoblasts. Corticosteroid-naïve DMD patients were compared with aged-matched controls and *mdx* mice were compared with wild-type mice. Differences observed in BMD between the *mdx* and wild-type mice were consistent with differences in BMD between DMD and control subjects. The investigators also identified increased populations of osteoclasts, RANKL/OPG ratio abnormalities that favored bone resorption, and significantly increased levels of IL-6, a recognized inhibitor of osteoblast function.

Vitamin D status in DMD
Because of the challenges previously described, vitamin D and calcium nutritional status are very difficult to analyze because quality data on normal vitamin D and calcium status in healthy children is limited. Nonetheless, it is clear that many boys with DMD are insufficient or deficient in vitamin D. Bianchi and colleagues[121] published a follow-up study of 33 children with DMD being treated with a fixed dose of prednisone (1.25 mg/kg every 2 days). Patients were observed for the first year and then treated with vitamin D_3 (0.8 μg/kg per day) plus adjustment of dietary calcium to the internationally recommended daily allowance for 2 additional years. During the observation year, BMC and BMD decreased in all patients. At the end of the 2-year supplementation phase, BMC and BMD significantly increased in more than 65% of patients. Bone metabolism parameters and BTMs were also reported to have normalized in most patients (78.8%). These results reveal important aspects about the bone disorder in DMD patients. Components of osteomalacia are suggested by observed improvement of low BMC and BMD with repletion of vitamin D. However, aspects of osteoporosis remain even after improved vitamin D and calcium nutritional status.

Amyotrophic Lateral Sclerosis

ALS is a rapidly progressive neurodegenerative disease caused by the loss of both upper and lower motor neurons throughout the neuraxis, including the motor cortex, brainstem, and spinal cord. The loss of motor neurons most typically results in a mixed picture of spasticity, diffuse muscular atrophy, and weakness. Most cases of ALS are presumably acquired and occur sporadically, with only about 10% occurring by familial inheritance.[137] The etiology of sporadic ALS is as yet unknown, but data suggests a multifactorial process ending in a final common pathway of motor-neuron apoptosis.[138] Familial and sporadic ALS cases are clinically indistinguishable.

ALS most commonly strikes individuals between the ages of 50 and 74 years, with a reported mean age of onset reported to extend from 58 to 63 years.[139–141] The incidence is approximately 1 to 3 per 100,000 with an overall prevalence rate of 5 to 10 per 100,000, making it one of the most common NMDs worldwide.[142,143] The 50% median survival rate is approximately 2 years after diagnosis.[139,141] Abnormalities in calcium metabolism have long been identified in ALS patients. In a retrospective study published in 1976, the investigators reviewed the records of 39 patients to discover that 20% had abnormal serum calcium levels and more than 50% showed radiographic evidence of bone abnormalities.[144] However, the literature regarding bone health in ALS remains very limited.

Fractures in ALS

Fractures occur commonly in ALS. Disease progression causes early discoordination and imbalance, which promotes an increased frequency of falls in patients as they approach the time of loss of independent mobility. In fact, in a multicenter clinical trial, falls were the third most common adverse event reported, and fall-related deaths have been reported to occur in 1.7% of ALS patients.[145,146] Several studies have found that fractures are more frequent among ALS patients than in controls. In the case-control study by Campbell,[4] ALS patients had 14% more fractures than controls. In a retrospective study, Kurtzke and Beebe[147] reviewed the military records of 504 men who died of ALS and found excess hospital admissions for trauma and fracture, particularly of the limbs and skull. The increased rate of fractures, skeletal abnormalities, and trauma in ALS patients was initially thought to be a risk factor for developing disease; however, further population studies investigating an association between trauma and ALS have not established a causal link, suggesting that these findings are more likely due to early prediagnostic symptoms of disease.[148–150]

In an attempt to lower the incidence of fractures in their ALS population, Sato and colleagues[151] treated 82 ALS patients, after random assignment, to daily treatment with 400 mg of etidronate or placebo over a 2-year period. At baseline, both groups had low BMD with high levels of serum ionized calcium and BTMs. In the etidronate group, serum calcium and marker levels decreased significantly during the study period, whereas the levels in the placebo group were increased. BMD decreased in all patients but was substantially slowed in the etidronate group compared with placebo (3.6% vs 12.1%; $P<.0001$). Fractures occurred in 7 patients in the placebo group and 1 patient in the risedronate group, with relative risk in the risedronate group in comparison with the placebo group of 0.14 (95% confidence interval, 0.02–1.11). These data suggest that there may be an opportunity to initiate early treatment directed at bone health, and perhaps avoid the morbidity associated with poor bone health and abnormal BMD in ALS.

BMD and vitamin D status in ALS

Few studies have evaluated bone density and markers of bone health in ALS. In addition to reducing fracture-related morbidity, there is an opportunity to examine the effects of an asymmetric progressive neurodegenerative disease on bone health in this unique patient population. With mounting evidence supporting a major role of the nervous system in bone metabolism, further studies may add to our understanding of the basic biological mechanisms involved in the maintenance of healthy bone. One small study examined the effects of chronic asymmetric neurologic impairment on bone density, evaluating patients with cerebrovascular disease (CVD), Parkinson disease (PD), and ALS. A high incidence of osteoporosis and right/left difference in osteopenia was reported. CVD and PD patients with asymmetric osteopenia showed an association between clinical symptoms, peripheral circulatory symptoms, and predominant osteopenia. Although the muscle strength of PD patients was reported as normal, the more severely affected side for PD symptoms and autonomic symptoms coincided with predominant osteopenia in the body. Increased bone resorption was detected in all ALS patients.[152]

In an earlier study, preceding their etidronate clinical trial, Sato and colleagues[153] assessed the bone health of 11 patients with ALS using bone density and serum biochemical indices of bone metabolism in a comparison with controls. The investigators identified vitamin D deficiency in 2 and insufficiency in 9 ALS patients. In addition, the mean serum 25-hydroxyvitamin D was significantly lower in ALS patients than in controls (14.0 ± 3.7 ng/mL vs 25.2 ± 4.0 ng/mL). Serum PTH and ionized calcium were elevated in 8 and 6 patients, respectively. z-Scores of metacarpal bone density were in the deficient range for 7 of the 11 ALS patients. These data underscore the potential importance of hypovitaminosis D and compensatory hyperparathyroidism in the development of osteopenia in patients with ALS.

In addition, as the general population ages and the ALS community identifies disease-slowing treatments, increasing the prevalence of patients with ALS, poor bone health will likely become a more frequent and thus a more costly problem, owing to fracture-related morbidity. Further studies are urgently needed to elucidate the prevalence of metabolic bone disease in ALS, determine the best diagnostic and treatment strategies, and evaluate the efficacy and timing of interventions. The potential to evaluate the contributions of nutritional (vitamin D), endocrine (parathyroid), and neurologic impairment and bone health–directed treatment in ALS, with its asymmetric, progressive disease course, is intriguing. Because of the complex nature of bone metabolism and maintenance, the implications of these studies may provide widespread benefits for patients with diverse causes of neurologic and neuromuscular disease, thus contributing to a better understanding of the basic pathology of bone disease.

Spinal Muscular Atrophy

There are several clinical presentations of SMA, all of which involve selective destruction of anterior horn cells. The various subtypes of SMA are clinically heterogeneous, with some rare forms affecting distal or bulbar muscles only. However, SMA usually has onset of symptoms in childhood and is inherited as an autosomal recessive trait. The incidence of SMA is about 1 in 10,000 live births with a carrier frequency of 1 in 50.[154]

The gene responsible for childhood-onset SMA has been mapped to chromosome 5q11.2-13.3. The causative gene, survival motor neuron 1 (SMN1), and a disease-modifying gene, survival motor neuron 2 (SMN2), have been identified. The most common abnormality of the SMN1 gene is a deletion of exon 7, but other exon deletions and point mutations can be disease causative. The SMN protein is ubiquitously expressed in all tissues, with high levels in the nervous system.[155,156] Recent data indicate that SMN1 deficiency alters stoichiometry of small nuclear ribonucleoproteins and leads to splicing defects for numerous genes in all cells, including motor neurons.[157]

The full-length transcripts of SMN1 and SMN2 encode proteins with an identical sequence; however, structural differences in the SMN2 gene cause frequent but not absolute exclusion of exon 7 during splicing.[158,159] The copy number of SMN2 varies in the population, and this variation appears to have important disease-modifying effects on SMA severity, with more SMN2 gene copies resulting in a less severe disease.[160]

The most common forms of SMA are often referred to as types I, II, and III.[161] SMA I is a severe disorder often resulting in death before 2 years of age, although longevity has been increased as a result of better medical management of disease sequelae.[162,163] Children with SMA I never attain the ability to sit independently. SMA II is less severe, with signs and symptoms becoming apparent in the first 18 months of life. These children sit independently but do not ambulate without assistance. SMA III has later onset, and all early developmental milestones including independent ambulation are acquired. In prior studies looking at SMA II and III over a 10-year period, SMA II subjects showed marked weakness and progressive decline of strength whereas SMA III subjects had less weakness and a relatively static, slowly progressive course. SMA III is consistent with a normal life span.[161]

Scoliosis in SMA

Similar to DMD, an early sign of poor bone health is the high prevalence of severe progressive scoliosis in SMA. Scoliosis, with increasing pelvic obliquity, is a common feature occurring in the early childhood of patients with SMA II (**Fig. 2**).[164] Several studies have been published documenting the incidence, severity, and progression of scoliosis, while comparing phenotypes and treatment outcomes.[165–167] Rodillo and colleagues[166] reviewed the incidence and severity of scoliosis in 37 patients with SMA II and 26 with SMA III. In SMA II, scoliosis had an early onset and rapid progression before puberty. The rapid progression occurred despite consistent use of a spinal brace, and spinal fusion was needed in all cases. In patients with SMA III, scoliosis was more variable. Scoliosis was present in 30% of patients and progressed rapidly during puberty in those who lost ambulation. Progression of scoliosis was slow in all who maintained ambulation, even if ambulation was assisted by

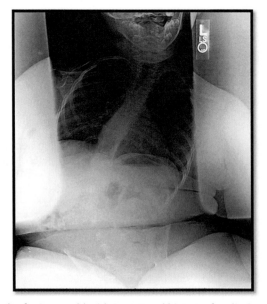

Fig. 2. A radiograph of a 6-year-old with SMA II and history of scoliosis, revealing a 61° dextroscoliotic curvature of the thoracolumbar spine.

orthoses. Granata and colleagues[167] reviewed 63 spinal radiographs of affected patients. All but one of the SMA II patients, and all of the SMA III patients who stopped ambulating had scoliosis, ranging from 10° to 165°. Of the 19 ambulatory SMA III patients 12 had scoliosis, ranging from 10° to 45°. Mean age at onset was 4 years 4 months in SMA II, and 9 years 10 months in SMA III. The severity of scoliosis in SMA has been reported to affect respiratory function, with a near linear inverse relationship to the patient's percent predicted forced vital capacity. With surgical correction, improvement in respiratory outcome measures have been observed, suggesting the potential of improved respiratory function if treatment-altering bone health is efficacious and reduces scoliosis severity.[168]

Fractures in SMA

Fractures are also common in this patient population, and fracture risk increases with severity of disease phenotype and loss of ambulation. The literature contains case reports describing congenital fractures in the most severe phenotypes of SMA.[169,170] The relative risk for fracture in SMA II and SMA III patients was 2.6 and 1.1, respectively when compared with age-matched controls in a study of 89 SMA patients.[115] In a questionnaire-based study, 9.3% of 93 respondents with SMA I, II, or III had previous fractures, of which those of the femur and humeral bones were most commonly reported.[5] A recently published retrospective study by Fujak and colleagues[171] supported the finding of increased prevalence of femur fractures in SMA patients. Of 131 patients, 60 (46%) suffered a total of 94 fractures. Most of the fractures (n = 50) were localized to the femur. Four SMA II patients suffered simultaneous fractures of both femurs, and one of these patients had sustained congenital femoral fractures.

BMD in SMA

Laboratory and animal studies have implicated the exon-7 splice variant of SMN as a participant in the upregulation of osteocyte-stimulatory factor, causing enhanced osteoclast formation and favoring bone resorption.[172] Osteoclast lineage cells were exposed to media from cells expressing the abnormal gene, and increased osteoclast formation occurred along with upregulation of mRNA involved in pathways regulating bone resorption. Animal studies, using the SMN2 mouse model of SMA, confirmed the role of SMN in bone remodeling using micro–computed tomography analysis of the lumbar vertebrae, tibia, and femurs. There was severely decreased BMD, and histologic evaluation of the bone tissue identified increased numbers of activated osteoclasts and upregulation of RANK-receptor signaling molecules critical for osteoclast differentiation.[173] Few human studies have evaluated BMD in SMA patients. However, results from a DXA study evaluating BMD in patients with varying NMD diagnoses, including a subset of patients with SMA, revealed the lowest BMD in the SMA cohort. The z-scores of the SMA patients were -2.25 ± 0.31, and nonambulatory SMA patients had significantly lower BMD compared with those who were still ambulatory ($P<.05$).[174]

Vitamin D status in SMA

The nutritional status and effectiveness of treatment using vitamin D in SMA patients has received very little attention. A PubMed literature search produced no related results. One study was identified through an online database search using Google Scholar, and was the research thesis of Alton[175] while enrolled at the University of Utah. Her study assessed 40 subjects with genetically confirmed SMA I, who were concurrently followed in a prospective natural history longitudinal study. Twenty-two males and 18 females with mean age of 18.6 months (range 0–165 months) were evaluated. Seventy-five percent of patients had inadequate intake of vitamin D at enrollment, in comparison with the American Academy of Pediatrics recommendation of 400 IU/d. Vitamin D and calcium intake were positively correlated with BMD and when increased, vitamin D and calcium consumption were associated with a significant increase in BMD as determined by whole-body DXA ($P = .04$ and $P = .01$, respectively).[175] These results suggest a potential role for vitamin D therapy in SMA, and highlight the urgent need for further well-designed prospective studies assessing vitamin D nutrition both with and without calcium supplementation.

SUMMARY

Bone disease is a significant problem for patients with neuromuscular disease. Bone density is frequently impaired and fracture risk is increased. The report of the patient with DMD or ALS who loses ambulation following a fracture is all too common. Studies evaluating potential bone-sparing therapies in the NMD patient population are few.

The pathophysiologic basis of each NMD may have its own unique effect on bone quality, as demonstrated by the literature regarding bone health in DMD, ALS, and SMA. Questions regarding these processes are unresolved. However, concomitant osteomalacia, secondary to vitamin D nutritional deficiency and abnormalities in PTH expression, are likely widespread and treatable. The gains in added bone mass through treatment, even without complete reversal of the bone defects, may be sufficient to slow bone loss, reduce fractures, and prolong ambulation.

In addition, the opportunity exists to capitalize on current discovery and pursue rational therapeutic strategies; for example, the potential role of β-blockade to improve bone mass in patients being treated with long-term glucocorticoids or who have nervous system disease, or the role of multinutrient therapy in neuromuscular-related bone disease, to name a few.

High-quality prospective studies using reliable biomarkers are needed to determine the prevalence of bone abnormalities and to define the best treatment strategies. In addition to improving the quality of life of NMD patients, these studies would present the opportunity to add to the knowledge base of the biology of bone health.

REFERENCES

1. Bone and joint initiative USA. Available at: http://www.usbji.org/. Accessed March 14, 2012.
2. Jacobs J, Anderssen G, Bell J, et al. An executive summary: the burden of musculoskeletal disease in the United States, prevalence, societal and economic cost. Available at: www.boneandjointburden.org. Accessed September 18, 2012.
3. Morgenroth VH, Hache LP, Clemens PR. Insights into bone health in Duchenne muscular dystrophy. BoneKEy Reports 2012.
4. Campbell AM. A survey of 190 cases of motor neurone disease. Riv Patol Nerv Ment 1965;86(2):211–7.
5. Granata C, Giannini S, Villa D, et al. Fractures in myopathies. Chir Organi Mov 1991;76:39–45.
6. Hadjidakis DJ, Androulakis II. Bone remodeling. Ann N Y Acad Sci 2006;1092: 385–96.
7. Kenny AM, Raisz LG. Mechanisms of bone remodeling: implications for clinical practice. J Reprod Med 2002;47(Suppl 1):63–70.
8. Adler CP. Bones and bone tissue; normal anatomy and histology. In: Claus-Peter A, editor. Bone diseases: Macroscopic, Histological, and Radiological Diagnosis of Structural Changes in the Skeleton. New York: Springer-Verlag; 2000. p. 1–30.

9. Ducy P, Desbois C, Boyce B, et al. Increased bone formation in osteocalcin-deficient mice. Nature 1996;382:448–52.

10. Luo G, Ducy P, Mckee MD, et al. Spontaneous calcification of arteries and cartilage in mice lacking matrix GLA protein. Nature 1997;386:78–81.

11. Xu T, Bianco P, Fisher LW, et al. Targeted disruption of the biglycan gene leads to an osteoporosis-like phenotype in mice. Nat Genet 1998;20:78–82.

12. Bachrach LK. Acquisition of optimal bone mass in childhood and adolescence. Trends Endocrinol Metab 2001;12:22–8.

13. Gilsanz V, Skaggs DL, Kovanlikaya A, et al. Differential effect of race on the axial and appendicular skeletons of children. J Clin Endocrinol Metab 1998;83: 1420–7.

14. Parfitt AM. Osteonal and hemi-osteonal remodeling: the spatial and temporal framework for signal traffic in adult human bone. J Cell Biochem 1994;55: 273–86.

15. Xiong J, O'Brien CA. Osteocyte RANKL: new insights into the control of bone remodeling. J Bone Miner Res 2012;27(3):499–505.

16. Suda T, Takahashi N, Udagawa N, et al. Modulation of osteoclast differentiation and function by the new members of the tumor necrosis factor receptor and ligand families. Endocr Rev 1999;20:345–57.

17. Hsu H, Lacey DL, Dunstan CR, et al. Tumor necrosis factor receptor family member RANK mediates osteoclast differentiation and activation induced by osteoprotegerin ligand. Proc Natl Acad Sci U S A 1999;96:3540–5.

18. Hofbauer LC, Schoppet M. Clinical implications of the osteoprotegerin/RANKL/RANK system for bone and vascular diseases. JAMA 2004;292:490–5.

19. Simonet WS, Lacey DL, Dunstan CR, et al. Osteoprotegerin: a novel secreted protein involved in the regulation of bone density. Cell 1997;89:309–19.

20. Karsenty G, Kronenberg HM, Settembre C. Genetic control of bone formation. Annu Rev Cell Dev Biol 2009;25:629–48.

21. Leucht P, Minear S, Ten Berge DR, et al. Translating insights from development into regenerative medicine: the function of Wnts in bone biology. Semin Cell Dev Biol 2008;19:434–43.

22. Krishnan V, Bryant HU, Macdougald OA. Regulation of bone mass by Wnt signaling. J Clin Invest 2006;116(5):1202–9.

23. Potts JT. Parathyroid hormone: past and present. J Endocrinol 2005;187:311–25.

24. Vilardaga JP, Romero G, Friedman PA, et al. Molecular basis of parathyroid hormone receptor signaling and trafficking: a family B GPCR paradigm. Cell Mol Life Sci 2010;68:1–13.

25. Taylor CW, Tovey SC. From parathyroid hormone to cytosolic Ca^{2+} signals. Biochem Soc Trans 2012;40(1):147–52.

26. Sato M, Westmore M, Ma YL, et al. Teriparatide [PTH(1–34)] strengthens the proximal femur of ovariectomized nonhuman primates despite increasing porosity. J Bone Miner Res 2004;19:623–9.

27. Ellegaard M, Jørgensen NR, Schwarz P. Parathyroid hormone and bone healing. Calcif Tissue Int 2010;87(1):1–13.

28. Pierroz DD, Bonnet N, Baldock PA, et al. Are osteoclasts needed for the bone anabolic response to parathyroid hormone? A study of intermittent parathyroid hormone with denosumab or alendronate in knock-in mice expressing humanized RANKL. J Biol Chem 2010;285(36):28164–73.

29. Tu PH, Liu ZH, Lee ST, et al. Treatment of repeated and multiple new-onset osteoporotic vertebral compression fractures with teriparatide. J Clin Neurosci 2012; 19(4):532–5.

30. Nicholson G, Moseley J, Sexton P, et al. Abundant calcitonin receptors in isolate rat osteoclasts, biochemical, and autoradiographic characterization. J Clin Invest 1986;78:355–60.

31. Manicourt DH, Azria M, Mindeholm L, et al. Oral salmon calcitonin reduces Lequesne's algofunctional index scores and decreases urinary and serum levels of biomarkers of joint metabolism in knee osteoarthritis. Arthritis Rheum 2006; 54(10):3205–11.

32. Clarke BL, Khosla S. Androgens and bone. Steroids 2009;74(3):296–305.

33. Vanderschueren D, Vandenput L, Boonen S, et al. Androgens and bone. Endocr Rev 2004;25:389–425.

34. Mauras N, Haymond MW, Darmaun D, et al. Calcium and protein kinetics in prepubertal boys. Positive effects of testosterone. J Clin Invest 1994;93:1014–9.

35. Behre HM, Kliesch S, Liefke E, et al. Long-term effect of testosterone therapy on bone mineral density in hypogonadal men. J Clin Endocrinol Metab 1997;82: 2386–90.

36. Carrascosa A, Audi L, Ferrandez MA, et al. Biological effects of androgens and identification of specific dihydrotestosterone-binding sites in cultured human fetal epiphyseal chondrocytes. J Clin Endocrinol Metab 1990;70:134–40.

37. Kerrigan JR, Rogol AD. The impact of gonadal steroid hormone action on growth hormone secretion during childhood and adolescence. Endocr Rev 1992;13:281–98.

38. Bord S, Horner A, Beavan S, et al. Estrogen receptors α and β are differentially expressed in developing human bone. J Clin Endocrinol Metab 2001;86:2309–14.

39. Nilsson LO, Boman A, Savendahl L, et al. Demonstration of estrogen receptor-β immunoreactivity in human growth plate cartilage. J Clin Endocrinol Metab 1999; 84:370–3.

40. Juul A. The effects of estrogens on linear bone growth. Hum Reprod Update 2001;7:303–13.

41. Falahati-Nini A, Riggs BL, Atkinson EJ, et al. Relative contributions of testosterone and estrogen in regulating bone resorption and formation in normal elderly men. J Clin Invest 2000;106:1553–60.

42. Leder BZ, LeBlanc KM, Schoenfeld DA, et al. Differential effects of androgens and estrogens on bone turnover in normal men. J Clin Endocrinol Metab 2003;88:204–10.

43. Riggs BL, Khosla S, Melton LJ. Sex steroids and the construction and conservation of the adult skeleton. Endocr Rev 2002;23:279–302.

44. Khosla S, Melton LJ, Riggs BL. Estrogen and the male skeleton. J Clin Endocrinol Metab 2002;87:1443–50.

45. Anderson FH, Francis RM, Faulkner K. Androgen supplementation in eugonadal men with osteoporosis: effects of 6 months of treatment on bone mineral density and cardiovascular risk factors. Bone 1996;18:171–7.

46. Chen H, Gilbert LC, Lu X, et al. New regulator of osteoclastogenesis: estrogen response element-binding protein in bone. J Bone Miner Res 2011;26(10): 2537–47.

47. Delany AM, Dong Y, Canalis E. Mechanisms of glucocorticoid action in bone cells. J Cell Biochem 1994;56(3):295–302.

48. Kalak R, Zhou H, Street J, et al. Endogenous glucocorticoid signalling in osteoblasts is necessary to maintain normal bone structure in mice. Bone 2009;45(1):61–7.

49. Zhou H, Mak W, Zheng Y, et al. Osteoblasts directly control lineage commitment of mesenchymal progenitor cells through Wnt signaling. J Biol Chem 2008;283: 1936–45.

50. Leclerc N, Luppen CA, Ho VV, et al. Gene expression profiling of glucocorticoid-inhibited osteoblasts. J Mol Endocrinol 2004;33:175–93.
51. Massafra U, Migliaccio S, Bancheri C, et al. Approach in glucocorticoid induced osteoporosis (GIO) prevention: results from the Italian multicenter observational EGEO study. J Endocrinol Invest 2012 [Abstract].
52. Canalis E, Delany AM. Mechanisms of glucocorticoid action in bone. Ann N Y Acad Sci 2002;966:73–81.
53. Manolagas SC, Weinstein RS. New developments in the pathogenesis and treatment of steroid-induced osteoporosis. J Bone Miner Res 1999;14:1061–6.
54. Weinstein RS. Glucocorticoid-induced osteoporosis. Rev Endocr Metab Disord 2001;2:65–73.
55. Kim HJ. New understanding of glucocorticoid action in bone cells. BMB Rep 2010;43(8):524–9.
56. Grossman JM, Gordon R, Ranganath VK, et al. American College of Rheumatology 2010 recommendations for the prevention and treatment of glucocorticoid-induced osteoporosis. Arthritis Care Res 2010;62(11):1515–26.
57. Bushby K, Finkel R, Birnkrant DJ, et al, DMD Care Considerations Working Group. Diagnosis and management of Duchenne muscular dystrophy, part 1: diagnosis, and pharmacological and psychosocial management. Lancet Neurol 2010;9(1):77–93.
58. Abe E, Sun L, Mechanick J, et al. Bone loss in thyroid disease: role of low TSH and high thyroid hormone. Ann N Y Acad Sci 2007;1116:383–91.
59. Williams GR. Actions of thyroid hormones in bone. Endokrynol Pol 2009;60(5): 380–8.
60. Gogakos AI, Duncan Bassett JH, Williams GR. Thyroid and bone. Arch Biochem Biophys 2010;503(1):129–36.
61. Xing W, Govoni K, Donahue LR, et al. Genetic evidence that thyroid hormone is indispensable for prepubertal IGF-I expression and bone acquisition in mice. J Bone Miner Res 2012 May;27(5):1067–79.
62. Serre CM, Farlay D, Delmas PD, et al. Evidence for a dense and intimate innervation of the bone tissue, including glutamate-containing fibers. Bone 1999; 25(6):623–9.
63. Takeda S. Central control of bone remodeling. J Neuroendocrinol 2008;20: 802–7.
64. Chenu C. Glutamatergic innervation in bone. Microsc Res Tech 2002;58(2):70–6.
65. Takeda S. Osteoporosis: a neuroskeletal disease? Int J Biochem Cell Biol 2009; 41(3):455–9.
66. Ahima RS, Flier JS. Leptin. Annu Rev Physiol 2000;62:413–37.
67. Ducy P, Amling M, Takeda S, et al. Leptin inhibits bone formation through a hypothalamic relay: a central control of bone mass. Cell 2000;100:197–207.
68. Elefteriou F, Ahn JD, Takeda S, et al. Leptin regulation of bone resorption by the sympathetic nervous system and CART. Nature 2005;434:514–20.
69. Takeda S, Elefteriou F, Levasseur R, et al. Leptin regulates bone formation via the sympathetic nervous system. Cell 2002;111:305–17.
70. Kajimura D, Hinoi E, Ferron M, et al. Genetic determination of the cellular basis of the sympathetic regulation of bone mass accrual. J Exp Med 2011;208(4): 841–51.
71. Ma Y, Nyman JS, Tao H, et al. β2-Adrenergic receptor signaling in osteoblasts contributes to the catabolic effect of glucocorticoids on bone. Endocrinology 2011;152(4):1412–22.

72. Mesías M, Seiquer I, Navarro MP. Calcium nutrition in adolescence. Crit Rev Food Sci Nutr 2011;51(3):195–209.

73. Wei MY, Giovannucci EL. Vitamin D and multiple health outcomes in the Harvard cohorts. Mol Nutr Food Res 2010;54(8):1114–26.

74. Lips P. Vitamin D physiology. Prog Biophys Mol Biol 2006;92(1):4–8.

75. Looker A, Mussolino M. Serum 25-hydroxyvitamin D and hip fracture risk in older U.S. white adults. J Bone Miner Res 2008;23:143–50.

76. DIPART (Vitamin D Individual Patient Analysis of Randomized Trials) Group. Patient level pooled analysis of 68,500 patients from seven major vitamin D fracture trials in US and Europe. BMJ 2010;340:b5463.

77. Tang BM, Eslick GD, Nowson C, et al. Use of calcium or calcium in combination with vitamin D supplementation to prevent fractures and bone loss in people aged 50 years and older: a meta-analysis. Lancet 2007;370:657–66.

78. Holick MF, Chen TC, Lu Z, et al. Vitamin D and skin physiology: a D-lightful story. J Bone Miner Res 2007;22:28–33.

79. Jones G. Pharmacokinetics of vitamin D toxicity. Am J Clin Nutr 2008;88:582–6.

80. Ross AC, Manson JE, Abrams SA, et al. The 2011 report on dietary reference intakes for calcium and vitamin D from the Institute of Medicine: what clinicians need to know. J Clin Endocrinol Metab 2011 Jan;96(1):52–8.

81. Gallagher JC, Sai A, Templin T 2nd, et al. Dose response to vitamin d supplementation in postmenopausal women: a randomized trial. Ann Intern Med 2012;156(6):425–37.

82. Heaney RP, Davies KM, Chen TC, et al. Human serum 25-hydroxycholecalciferol response to extended oral dosing with cholecalciferol. Am J Clin Nutr 2003;77: 204–10.

83. Hanley DA, Cranney A, Jones G, et al, Guidelines Committee of the Scientific Advisory Council of Osteoporosis Canada. Vitamin D in adult health and disease: a review and guideline statement from Osteoporosis Canada (summary). CMAJ 2010;182(12):1315–9.

84. Institute of Medicine. Dietary reference intakes for calcium, phosphorus, magnesium, vitamin D and fluoride. Washington, DC: National Academy Press; 1997.

85. Lai JK, Lucas RM, Clements MS, et al. Assessing vitamin D status: pitfalls for the unwary. Mol Nutr Food Res 2010;54(8):1062–71.

86. Lai JK, Lucas RM, Banks E, et al, Ausimmune Investigator Group. Variability in vitamin D assays impairs clinical assessment of vitamin D status. Intern Med J 2012;42(1):43–50.

87. Weber P. Vitamin K and bone health. Nutrition 2001;17(10):880–7.

88. Kanellakis S, Moschonis G, Tenta R, et al. Changes in parameters of bone metabolism in postmenopausal women following a 12-month intervention period using dairy products enriched with calcium, vitamin D, and phylloquinone (vitamin K(1)) or menaquinone-7 (vitamin K (2)): the postmenopausal health study II. Calcif Tissue Int 2012;90(4):251–62.

89. Rude RK, Singer FR, Gruber HE. Skeletal and hormonal effects of magnesium deficiency. J Am Coll Nutr 2009;28(2):131–41.

90. Genuis SJ, Bouchard TP. Combination of micronutrients for bone (COMB) study: bone density after micronutrient intervention. J Environ Public Health 2012;2012: 354151.

91. Kohrt WM, Bloomfield SA, Little KD, et al. American College of Sports Medicine position stand on physical activity and bone health. Med Sci Sports Exerc 2004; 36:1985–96.

92. Heaney RP, Abrams S, Dawson-Hughes B, et al. Peak bone mass. Osteoporos Int 2000;11:985–1009.
93. Lanyon LE, Rubin CT. Static vs dynamic loads as an influence on bone remodeling. J Biomech 1984;17:897–905.
94. Martyn-St James M, Carroll SJ. Effects of different impact exercise modalities on bone mineral density in premenopausal women: a meta-analysis. Bone Miner Metab 2010;28(3):251–67.
95. Takata S, Yasui N. Disuse osteoporosis. J Med Invest 2001;48(3–4):147–56.
96. Rittweger J, Simunic B, Bilancio G, et al. Bone loss in the lower leg during 35 days of bed rest is predominantly from the cortical compartment. Bone 2009;44(4):612–8.
97. Garland DE, Stewart CA, Adkins RH, et al. Osteoporosis after spinal cord injury. J Orthop Res 1992;10(3):371–8.
98. Reyes ML, Hernández M, Holmgren LJ, et al. High-frequency, low-intensity vibrations increase bone mass and muscle strength in upper limbs, improving autonomy in disabled children. J Bone Miner Res 2011;26(8):1759–66.
99. Tezval M, Biblis M, Sehmisch S, et al. Improvement of femoral bone quality after low-magnitude, high-frequency mechanical stimulation in the ovariectomized rat as an osteopenia model. Calcif Tissue Int 2011;88(1):33–40.
100. Engelke K, Adams J, Armbrecht G. Clinical use of quantitative computed tomography and peripheral quantitative computed tomography in the management of osteoporosis in adults: the 2007 ISCD official positions. J Clin Densitom 2008;11:123–62.
101. Leonard M, Bachrach L. Assessment of bone mineralization following renal transplantation in children: limitations of DXA and the confounding effects of delayed growth and development. Am J Transplant 2001;1:193–6.
102. Zemel BS, Kalkwarf HJ, Gilsanz V, et al. Revised reference curves for bone mineral content and areal bone mineral density according to age and sex for black and non-black children: results of the bone mineral density in childhood study. J Clin Endocrinol Metab 2011;96(10):3160–9.
103. Clark EM, Ness AR, Bishop NJ, et al. Association between bone mass and fractures in children: a prospective cohort study. J Bone Miner Res 2006;21:1489–95.
104. Lewiecki EM. Benefits and limitations of bone mineral density and bone turnover markers to monitor patients treated for osteoporosis. Curr Osteoporos Rep 2010;8(1):15–22.
105. Maybarduk PK, Levine M. Osseous atrophy associated with progressive muscular dystrophy. Am J Dis Child 1941;61:565–76.
106. Hsu JD. Extremity fractures in children with neuromuscular disease. Johns Hopkins Med J 1979;145:89–93.
107. Hsu JD. Skeletal changes in children with neuromuscular disorders. Prog Clin Biol Res 1982;101:553–7.
108. Drousiotou A, Ioannou P, Georgiou T, et al. Neonatal screening for Duchenne muscular dystrophy: a novel semiquantitative application of the bioluminescence test for creatine kinase in a pilot national program in Cyprus. Genet Test 1998;2:55–60.
109. Emery AE. Population frequencies of inherited neuromuscular diseases– a world survey. Neuromuscul Disord 1991;1:19–29.
110. Hoffman EP, Brown RH Jr, Kunkel LM. Dystrophin: the protein product of the Duchenne muscular dystrophy locus. Cell 1987;51:919–28.

111. Bushby K, Finkel R, Birnkrant DJ, et al, DMD Care Considerations Working Group. Diagnosis and management of Duchenne muscular dystrophy, part 2: implementation of multidisciplinary care. Lancet Neurol 2010;9:177–89.

112. Hatano E, Masuda K, Kameo H. Fractures in Duchenne muscular dystrophy—chiefly about their causes. Hiroshima J Med Sci 1986;35:429–33.

113. Siegel IM. Fractures of long bones in Duchenne muscular dystrophy. J Trauma 1977;17:219–22.

114. Larson CM, Henderson RC. Bone mineral density and fractures in boys with Duchenne muscular dystrophy. J Pediatr Orthop 2000;20(1):71–4.

115. Vestergaard P, Glerup H, Steffensen BF, et al. Fracture risk in patients with muscular dystrophy and spinal muscular atrophy. J Rehabil Med 2001;33(4): 150–5.

116. Aparicio LF, Jurkovic M, DeLullo J. Decreased bone density in ambulatory patients with Duchenne muscular dystrophy. J Pediatr Orthop 2002;22:179–81.

117. Talim B, Malaguti C, Gnudi S, et al. Vertebral compression in Duchenne muscular dystrophy following deflazacort. Neuromuscul Disord 2002;12:294–5.

118. McDonald DG, Kinali M, Gallagher AC, et al. Fracture prevalence in Duchenne muscular dystrophy. Dev Med Child Neurol 2002;44:695–8.

119. Bothwell JE, Gordon KE, Dooley JM, et al. Vertebral fractures in boys with Duchenne muscular dystrophy. Clin Pediatr (Phila) 2003;42:353–6.

120. Louis M, Lebacq J, Poortmans JR, et al. Beneficial effects of creatine supplementation in dystrophic patients. Muscle Nerve 2003;27:604–10.

121. Bianchi ML, Mazzanti A, Galbiati E, et al. Bone mineral density and bone metabolism in Duchenne muscular dystrophy. Osteoporos Int 2003;14:761–7.

122. Douvillez B, Braillon P, Hodgkinson I, et al. Pain, osteopenia and body composition of 22 patients with Duchenne muscular dystrophy: a descriptive study. Ann Readapt Med Phys 2005;48:616–22.

123. Hawker GA, Ridout R, Harris VA, et al. Alendronate in the treatment of low bone mass in steroid-treated boys with Duchenne's muscular dystrophy. Arch Phys Med Rehabil 2005;86:284–8.

124. Biggar WD, Politano L, Harris VA, et al. Deflazacort in Duchenne muscular dystrophy: a comparison of two different protocols. Neuromuscul Disord 2004; 14:476–82.

125. Biggar WD, Harris VA, Eliasoph L, et al. Long-term benefits of deflazacort treatment for boys with Duchenne muscular dystrophy in their second decade. Neuromuscul Disord 2006;16:249–55.

126. Bachrach LK. Taking steps towards reducing osteoporosis in Duchenne muscular dystrophy. Neuromuscul Disord 2005;15:86–7.

127. Biggar WD, Bachrach LK, Henderson RC, et al. Bone health in Duchenne muscular dystrophy: a workshop report from the meeting in Cincinnati, Ohio, July 8, 2004. Neuromuscul Disord 2005;15:80–5.

128. Quinlivan R, Roper H, Davie M, et al. Report of a muscular dystrophy campaign funded workshop Birmingham, UK, January 16th 2004. Osteoporosis in Duchenne muscular dystrophy; its prevalence, treatment and prevention. Neuromuscul Disord 2005;15:72–9.

129. Muntoni F, Bushby K, Manzur AY. Muscular dystrophy campaign funded workshop on management of scoliosis in Duchenne muscular dystrophy, 24 January 2005, London, UK. Neuromuscul Disord 2006;16:210–9.

130. Quinlivan R, Shaw N, Bushby K. 170th ENMC International Workshop: bone protection for corticosteroid treated Duchenne muscular dystrophy. 27-29

November 2009, Naarden, The Netherlands. Neuromuscul Disord 2010;20(11): 761–9.

131. Pecak F, Trontelj JV, Dimitrijevic MR. Scoliosis in neuromuscular disorders. Int Orthop 1980;3:323–8.

132. King WM, Ruttencutter R, Nagaraja HN, et al. Orthopedic outcomes of long-term daily corticosteroid treatment in Duchenne muscular dystrophy. Neurology 2007;68(19):1607–13.

133. Houde S, Filiatrault M, Fournier A, et al. Deflazacort use in Duchenne muscular dystrophy: an 8-year follow-up. Pediatr Neurol 2008;38:200–6.

134. Palmieri GM, Bertorini TE, Griffin JW, et al. Assessment of whole body composition with dual energy x-ray absorptiometry in Duchenne muscular dystrophy: correlation of lean body mass with muscle function. Muscle Nerve 1996;19: 777–9.

135. Söderpalm AC, Magnusson P, Åhlander AC, et al. Bone mass development in patients with Duchenne and Becker muscular dystrophies: a 4-year clinical follow-up. Acta Paediatr 2012;101(4):424–32.

136. Rufo A, Del Fattore A, Capulli M, et al. Mechanisms inducing low bone density in Duchenne muscular dystrophy in mice and humans. J Bone Miner Res 2011; 26(8):1891–903.

137. Siddique T, Deng H. Genetics of amyotrophic lateral sclerosis. Hum Mol Genet 1996;5(Spec No):1465–70.

138. Wijesekera LC, Leigh PN. Amyotrophic lateral sclerosis. Orphanet J Rare Dis 2009;4:3.

139. Norris F, Sheperd R, Denys E, et al. Onset, natural history and outcome in idiopathic adult motor neuron disease. J Neurol Sci 1993;118(1):48–55.

140. Pradas J, Finison L, Andres PL, et al. The natural history of amyotrophic lateral sclerosis and the use of natural history controls in therapeutic trials. Neurology 1993;43(4):751–5.

141. Ringel SP, Murphy JR, Alderson MK, et al. The natural history of amyotrophic lateral sclerosis. Neurology 1993;43(7):1316–22.

142. Huisman MH, de Jong SW, van Doormaal PT, et al. Population based epidemiology of amyotrophic lateral sclerosis using capture-recapture methodology. J Neurol Neurosurg Psychiatry 2011;82(10):1165–70. http://dx.doi.org/10.1136/jnnp.2011.244939.

143. Chancellor AM, Warlow CP. Adult onset motor neuron disease: worldwide mortality, incidence, and distribution since 1950. J Neurol Neurosurg Psychiatry 1992;55(12):1106–15.

144. Patten BM, Mallette LE. Motor neuron disease: retrospective study of associated abnormalities. Dis Nerv Syst 1976;37(6):318–21.

145. Montes J, Cheng B, Diamond B, et al. The timed up and go test: predicting falls in ALS. Amyotroph Lateral Scler 2007;8(5):292–5.

146. Aggarwal SP, Zinman L, Simpson E, et al, Northeast and Canadian Amyotrophic Lateral Sclerosis Consortia. Safety and efficacy of lithium in combination with riluzole for treatment of amyotrophic lateral sclerosis: a randomized double-blind, placebo-controlled trial. Lancet Neurol 2010;9:481–8.

147. Kurtzke JF, Beebe GW. Epidemiology of amyotrophic lateral sclerosis: 1. A case-control comparison based on ALS deaths. Neurology 1980;30(5):453–62.

148. Beghi E, Logroscino G, Chiò A, et al. Amyotrophic lateral sclerosis, physical exercise, trauma and sports: results of a population-based pilot case-control study. Amyotroph Lateral Scler 2010;11(3):289–92.

149. Strickland D, Smith SA, Dolliff G, et al. Physical activity, trauma, and ALS: a case-control study. Acta Neurol Scand 1996;94(1):45–50.

150. Cruz DC, Nelson LM, McGuire V, et al. Physical trauma and family history of neurodegenerative diseases in amyotrophic lateral sclerosis: a population-based case-control study. Neuroepidemiology 1999;18(2):101–10.

151. Sato Y, Honda Y, Iwamoto J. Etidronate for fracture prevention in amyotrophic lateral sclerosis: a randomized controlled trial. Bone 2006;39(5):1080–6.

152. Ishizaki F, Koyama T, Sunayashiki T, et al. Control of bone remodeling by nervous system. Bone metabolic changes in neurological diseases. Clin Calcium 2010;20(12):1841–9.

153. Sato Y, Honda Y, Asoh T, et al. Hypovitaminosis D and decreased bone mineral density in amyotrophic lateral sclerosis. Eur Neurol 1997;37(4):225–9.

154. Ogino S, Leonard DG, Rennert H, et al. Genetic risk assessment in carrier testing for spinal muscular atrophy. Am J Med Genet 2002;110(4):301–7.

155. Brzustowicz LM, Lehner T, Castilla LH, et al. Genetic mapping of chronic childhood-onset spinal muscular atrophy to chromosome 5Q11.2-13.3. Nature 1990;344:540–1.

156. Battaglia G, Princivalle A, Forti F, et al. Expression of the SMN gene, the spinal muscular atrophy determining gene, in the mammalian central nervous system. Hum Mol Genet 1997;6:1961–71.

157. Zhang Z, Lotti F, Dittmar K, et al. SMN deficiency causes tissue-specific perturbations in the repertoire of snRNAs and widespread defects in splicing. Cell 2008;133:585–600.

158. Boda B, Mas C, Giudicelli C, et al. Survival motor neuron SMN1 and SMN2 gene promoters: identical sequences and differential expression in neurons and non-neuronal cells. Eur J Hum Genet 2004;12(9):729–37.

159. Wirth B, Brichta L, Schrank B, et al. Mildly affected patients with spinal muscular atrophy are partially protected by an increased SMN2 copy number. Hum Genet 2006;119(4):422–8.

160. Swoboda KJ, Prior TW, Scott CB, et al. Natural history of denervation in SMA: relation to age, SMN2 copy number, and function. Ann Neurol 2005;57(5):704–12.

161. Carter GT, Abresch RT, Fowler WM, et al. Profiles of neuromuscular disease: spinal muscular atrophy. Am J Phys Med Rehabil 1995;74(5):S150–9.

162. Manna MM, Kalra M, Wong B, et al. Survival probabilities of patients with childhood spinal muscle atrophy. J Clin Neuromuscul Dis 2009;10(3):85–9.

163. MacKenzie AE, Jacob P, Surh L, et al. Genetic heterogeneity in spinal muscular atrophy: a link age analysis-based assessment. Neurology 1994;44:919–24.

164. Fujak A, Ingenhorst A, Heuser K, et al. Treatment of scoliosis in intermediate spinal muscular atrophy (SMA type II) in childhood. Ortop Traumatol Rehabil 2005;7(2):175–9.

165. Merlini L, Granata C, Bonfiglioli S, et al. Scoliosis in spinal muscular atrophy: natural history and management. Dev Med Child Neurol 1989;31(4):501–8.

166. Rodillo E, Marini ML, Heckmatt JZ, et al. Scoliosis in spinal muscular atrophy: review of 63 cases. J Child Neurol 1989;4(2):118–23.

167. Granata C, Merlini L, Magni E, et al. Spinal muscular atrophy: natural history and orthopaedic treatment of scoliosis. Spine 1989;14(7):760–2.

168. Robinson D, Galasko CS, Delaney C, et al. Scoliosis and lung function in spinal muscular atrophy. Eur Spine J 1995;4(5):268–73.

169. Felderhoff-Mueser U, Grohmann K, Harder A, et al. Severe spinal muscular atrophy variant associated with congenital bone fractures. J Child Neurol 2002;17(9):718–21.

170. Shanmugarajan S, Swoboda KJ, Iannaccone ST, et al. Congenital bone fractures in spinal muscular atrophy: functional role for SMN protein in bone remodeling. J Child Neurol 2007;22(8):967–73.
171. Fujak A, Kopschina C, Forst R, et al. Fractures in proximal spinal muscular atrophy. Arch Orthop Trauma Surg 2010;130(6):775–80.
172. Kurihara N, Menaa C, Maeda H, et al. Osteoclast-stimulating factor interacts with the spinal muscular atrophy gene product to stimulate osteoclast formation. J Biol Chem 2001;276(44):41035–9.
173. Shanmugarajan S, Tsuruga E, Swoboda KJ, et al. Bone loss in survival motor neuron (Smn(-/-) SMN2) genetic mouse model of spinal muscular atrophy. J Pathol 2009;219(1):52–60.
174. Khatri IA, Chaudhry US, Seikaly MG, et al. Low bone mineral density in spinal muscular atrophy. J Clin Neuromuscul Dis 2008;10(1):11–7.
175. Alton J. Prevalence of inadequate vitamin D intake in spinal muscular atrophy type I population as is correlates with bone health. University of Utah; 2011. Available at: http://gateway.proquest.com/openurl%3furl_ver=Z39.88-2004%26res_dat=xri:pqdiss%26rft_val_fmt=info:ofi/fmt:kev:mtx:dissertation%26rft_dat=xri:pqdiss:1493416. Accessed March 14, 2012.

Current Pharmacologic Management in Selected Neuromuscular Diseases

Andrew J. Skalsky, MD[a],*, Bjorn Oskarsson, MD[b], Jay J. Han, MD[c],
David Richman, MD[b]

KEYWORDS

- Amyotrophic lateral sclerosis • Myasthenia gravis • Inflammatory myopathy
- Myotonia • Spinal muscular atrophy • Duchenne muscular dystrophy

KEY POINTS

- Pompe disease is a heterogeneous hereditary neuromuscular disorder with an effective treatment.
- Riluzole remains the only disease-modifying treatment for amyotrophic lateral sclerosis (ALS) that is approved by the Food and Drug Administration; however, readily available symptomatic treatments can provide relief from the often-distressing symptoms associated with ALS and improve quality of life for the patient.
- Autoimmune inflammatory myopathies, except inclusion body myositis, characteristically respond with rapid improvement after the initiation of corticosteroid treatment.
- Treatments available for the neuromuscular junction disorders vary based on the underlying genetic or autoimmune abnormality, and should be individualized to avoid significant adverse events and provide the most efficacious disease management.
- New and promising gene-based drug therapies for Duchenne muscular dystrophy and spinal muscular atrophy are currently in clinical trial.

INTRODUCTION

Neuromuscular disorders are a collection of well-defined acquired or inherited clinical conditions that affect neuromuscular function. The clinical conditions are a highly heterogeneous group that can affect skeletal muscle, motor neurons, peripheral nerves, and neuromuscular junctions. In the past few decades, there has been a significant increase in the understanding of the pathophysiology of neuromuscular

[a] Department of Pediatrics, Rady Children's Hospital San Diego, University of California San Diego, 3020 Children's Way, San Diego, CA 92123, USA; [b] Department of Neurology, University of California Davis, 4860 Y Street, Suite 0100, Sacramento, CA 95817, USA; [c] Department of Physical Medicine and Rehabilitation, 4860 Y Street, Sacramento, CA 95817, USA
* Corresponding author.
E-mail address: askalsky@rchsd.org

Phys Med Rehabil Clin N Am 23 (2012) 801–820
http://dx.doi.org/10.1016/j.pmr.2012.09.003
1047-9651/12/$ – see front matter © 2012 Elsevier Inc. All rights reserved.

disorders whether attributable to a genetic etiology or an autoimmune process. With the better understanding of disease mechanisms leading to neuromuscular weakness, researchers have attempted to develop therapeutic interventions directly affecting the pathophysiology of the various disorders. Although the development of therapeutic interventions has been slow, the potential for significant therapeutic modalities remains promising.

PHARMACOLOGIC MANAGEMENT OF POMPE DISEASE

Pompe disease, also referred to as acid maltase deficiency (or glycogen storage disease type II), is a rare autosomal recessive disorder caused by deficiency of the glycogen-degrading lysosomal enzyme acid alpha-glucosidase (GAA).[1–6] Lysosomal GAA catalyzes the breakdown of glycogen into glucose, and the GAA deficiency in Pompe disease results in the accumulation of lysosomal and nonlysosomal glycogen in multiple tissues.[7–9] In the infantile-onset form of Pompe disease, GAA enzyme activity is either completely or nearly completely absent (typically <1% of normal activity). Some residual enzyme activity (approximately 2%–40% of normal activity) is present in most children and adults with the late-onset form.[10,11] Infantile-onset Pompe disease is a progressive, multisystemic disorder that causes hypotonia, cardiomyopathy, respiratory deficiency, and feeding difficulties in the first year of life. The disease affects cardiac, skeletal, and smooth muscles and the pulmonary and gastrointestinal systems, as well as anterior horn cells. Death owing to cardiopulmonary failure typically occurs in the first year of life, with rare survival past 2 years.[2,12] Late-onset Pompe disease is also a multisystemic disease; it may manifest at any time after 12 months of age. Its clinical presentation includes progressive muscle weakness, especially in the trunk and lower limbs; respiratory symptoms with restrictive lung disease pattern; and progression to respiratory insufficiency because of diaphragmatic and intercostal muscle involvement. Respiratory complications are the most frequent cause of death in the late-onset Pompe disease.

Alglucosidase Alfa

Disease-specific enzyme replacement treatment (ERT) strategy for Pompe disease was first attempted in 1973.[13] Highly purified, placenta-derived GAA enzyme was administered by intravenous infusion, taking advantage of the lysosome's ability to internalize exogenously delivered proteins by endocytosis. Initial attempts at ERT encountered problems of immunogenicity, and there was limited availability of purified GAA for practical and sustainable enzyme delivery.[13,14] In 1979, the 28-kb gene for GAA was identified on chromosome 17,[15] and in the 1990s, new recombinant DNA technology became available, enabling the production of enough recombinant human acid alpha-glucosidase (rhGAA) to allow ERT clinical trials to be conducted. In 2006, alglucosidase alfa (MYOZYME, Genzyme Corporation, Cambridge, MA)[16] was approved by the US Food and Drug Administration (FDA) and the European Medicines Agency and became the first disease-specific treatment for Pompe disease. The approval was based on the results of a pivotal clinical trial of ERT with alglucosidase alfa in 18 infants showing significant benefit.[17] The ERT with rhGAA improved ventilator-free survival, cardiomyopathy, growth, and motor function in patients with infantile-onset Pompe disease compared with outcomes expected for patients without treatment.

The results of the first randomized, double-blind, placebo-controlled study of ERT, known as the Late-Onset Treatment Study (LOTS),[18] led to the FDA approval in 2010 of LUMIZYME (Genzyme Corporation)[19] for the treatment of late-onset Pompe disease in the United States. Those who qualified for the study were randomly assigned in a ratio of 2:1 to receive biweekly infusions of alglucosidase alfa (20 mg/kg, based on body weight) or placebo. The LOTS trial was conducted in 90 patients 8 years or older (range, 10–70 years). The 2 coprimary end points were distance walked during a 6-minute walk test (6MWT) and the percent of predicted forced vital capacity (FVC) in the upright position. At week 78, statistically significant findings in favor of alglucosidase alfa were noted in both the 6MWT and percentage of predicted upright FVC results. All of the secondary and tertiary end points favored the treatment group, but only the MEP results reached statistical significance.[18] Similar frequencies of adverse events, serious adverse events, and treatment-related adverse events occurred in patients in both the treatment and placebo groups. Anaphylactic reactions occurred only in patients receiving ERT (5%, 3 of 60 treated). All of the alglucosidase alfa recipients tested negative for immunoglobulin G (IgG) anti-GAA antibodies at start of the trial, but all seroconverted by week 12. The study findings indicate that alglucosidase alfa has a positive effect on the disease process or processes that produce impaired ambulation and respiratory insufficiency in late-onset Pompe disease, but treatment carries a risk of serious potential complications, including anaphylactic reactions.[18,19] Because 5% of patients in the treatment group of the LOTS trial developed an anaphylactic reaction, caution is recommended during home-based infusion and patients treated with alglucosidase alfa who have persistently high antibody titers should be closely monitored until the effect of the antibodies is more fully understood.[20] Several treatment recommendation guidelines for Pompe disease are available.[21]

In the United States, LUMIZYME is available only through a restricted distribution program: the LUMIZYME ACE (Alglucosidase Alfa Control and Education) Program.[22] The program is a risk evaluation and mitigation strategy program designed to mitigate the potential risk of rapid disease progression in patients with infantile-onset Pompe disease and patients with late-onset disease who are younger than 8 years, for whom the safety and efficacy of LUMIZYME have not been evaluated in randomized, controlled studies. The LUMIZYME ACE Program acts to ensure that "the known risks of anaphylaxis and severe allergic reactions associated with the use of alglucosidase alfa are communicated to patients and prescribers and to ensure that potential risks of severe cutaneous and systemic immune-mediated reactions to alglucosidase alfa are communicated to patients and prescribers." Moreover, prescribers, health care facilities, and patients treated in the United States must enroll in the LUMIZYME ACE Program before alglucosidase alfa will be authorized for shipment, and prescribers and health care facilities at which ERT infusions will be conducted must complete the LUMIZYME ACE Program online certification (www.lumizyme.com/ace/default. asp).

The completion and successes of the infantile and late-onset Pompe trial with subsequent FDA approval of ERT as treatment for Pompe disease are tremendous achievements. Much work remains to be completed, however, including more basic research improving our understanding of the links between GAA enzyme deficiency, glycogen deposition, lysosomal function, and the various phenotypic presentations. For the future, other potential therapeutic approaches are also being explored that include small molecule pharmacologic chaperones, gene therapy (adeno-associated virus), and new-generation ERT with improved targeted delivery capabilities.

PHARMACOLOGIC MANAGEMENT OF AMYOTROPHIC LATERAL SCLEROSIS

Amyotrophic lateral sclerosis (ALS) remains a challenging condition to treat, and current medical treatments have only a modest effect on disease progression. ALS progressively causes muscle weakness and eventually respiratory failure. Mechanical ventilation can prolong life significantly, but this option is rarely used in North America because of patient preferences and sometimes because of economic concerns. The nonpharmacologic interventions of noninvasive ventilation and gastrostomy tubes provide prolonged life expectancy.

Riluzole

The only medication proven to slow ALS is riluzole. Its major pharmacologic effect in ALS is serving as a glutamate receptor blocker, thereby preventing excitotoxicity.[23] The medication also has a sodium channel blocking effect of uncertain relevance to ALS.[24] Riluzole has a modest benefit in animal models of ALS.[25] In human trials, survival was prolonged by 2 to 3 months.[26,27] Riluzole has failed to demonstrate any benefits on strength or breathing function. The modest survival benefit that has been demonstrated was shown in patients in a relatively early stage of disease and a trial of patients with more advanced disease did not demonstrate a survival advantage with riluzole. Patients with more advanced disease may not benefit from the medication or the benefit was too small to be detected in the trial of 168 patients.[28] Despite riluzole's clear effect on patients with early ALS, the drug is not uniformly used in North America, with only 59% of patients taking the drug.[29]

Riluzole is dosed at 50 mg daily for the first week and then 2 times daily thereafter. Elevated liver enzymes occurs 2.62 times more often in patients taking riluzole versus placebo.[30] Monitoring liver enzymes is advisable before treatment and after 1 month, followed by testing every 3 to 6 months. More common limiting side effects include gastrointestinal discomfort and diarrhea. Riluzole binds to food in the stomach. To ensure maximal absorption, it should be administered apart from meals.

Experimental Pharmacologic Management in ALS

Investigative approaches in early development are covered in a separate article in this issue. Currently there are 2 drugs in phase III trials in the United States: ceftriaxone and dexpramipexole. Both trials will be completed in late 2012. Ceftriaxone is a third-generation cephalosporin that was selected for the treatment of ALS through in vitro screening of available pharmacologic agents.[31] The effect of ceftriaxone pertinent to slowing disease progression in ALS is the upregulation of EAAT2, a glutamate transporter that protects neurons from excitotoxicity. Dexpramipexole is the dextro isomer of pramipexole, and it lacks the racemic pramipexole's strong dopaminergic effect. The lack of dopaminergic effect makes the drug tolerable at a many fold higher dose. Dexpramipexole has been shown to be neuroprotective in several animal models. A phase II trial in ALS done in 2008 was encouraging, suggesting a slowing of disease progression by 20%.[32]

Pharmacologic Management of Pseudobulbar Affect in ALS

Pseudobulbar affect (PBA) is a symptom that is experienced in about half of patients with ALS.[33] The term refers to a disconnect between emotion and affect that manifests as brief paroxysms of crying or laughing that is out of proportion, or sometimes even opposite, to the experienced emotion. Multiple other names, such as "inappropriate emotional expressive disorder" or "pathologic laughing and crying" and "emotional incontinence" have been proposed for the symptom because PBA is a term that does not describe the symptom.[34] There are several medications used to treat PBA symptoms. Dextromethorphan has the best evidence base with several studies showing an effect in ALS.[35] Dextromethorphan has to be combined with quinidine, which blocks its CYP450 2D6 breakdown to achieve an effective pharmacologic profile. Quinidine also leads to increased plasma levels of other drugs that are metabolized by the CYP450 2D6, but the drug combination otherwise has few side effects. Tricyclic antidepressants (TCAs) are also effective, and in particular amitriptyline with its strong anticholinergic effect is widely used for several indications in ALS care.[36] Last, the selective serotonin reuptake inhibitors (SSRIs) can also be effective, but anecdotally, they are the less effective than dextromethorphan and amitriptyline.

Pharmacologic Management of Symptoms in ALS

Dementia
Dementia or less severe cognitive deficits and behavioral changes occur in about half of patients with ALS,[37] but we lack pharmacologic treatments for the problem. The frontal lobe dysfunction seen in ALS is not helped by a centrally acting reversible acetylcholinesterase inhibitor like donepezil or by N-methyl-D-aspartate receptor blockers like memantine.

Fatigue
Fatigue is another common ALS symptom. Patients may experience low energy level and loss of stamina, often with daytime sleepiness, and difficulty concentrating. Nonpharmacologic management with energy conservation and noninvasive ventilation are useful, but pharmacologic agents can also be used. Modafinil has shown preliminary benefit in improving fatigue in ALS.[38] Modafinil can worsen anxiety, but no other side effects are common. Other options include activating SSRIs, such as fluoxetine, which also are effective against depression, anxiety, and PBA and may even help with weight maintenance.

Depression
Depression is not more common in ALS than in the general population, but it is a problem for a minority of ALS patients. Nonpharmacologic interventions, such as counseling and support groups, can help, but often an antidepressant is indicated. SSRI medications are normally the first-line agent against depression. The doses of TCA used to control other ALS symptoms are generally insufficient to have an effect on depression.

Anxiety
Anxiety often relates to specific fears regarding dying and terminal symptoms, such as shortness of breath. Information and discussion of specific fears can often very effectively alleviate anxiety. When information and reassurance are not enough, then the SSRIs are again useful and form the mainstay of preventive treatment. Benzodiazepines are very effective in acutely reducing anxiety, and also help spasticity and muscle cramps. Benzodiazepines reduce respiratory drive, which can result in respiratory depression and carbon dioxide retention. Patients with near normal breathing function are not at an increased risk of developing respiratory depression, but this does become a major concern as respiratory function decreases. Ventilated patients do not suffer in the same way from depression of respiratory drive, and noninvasive positive pressure ventilation does at least partially address the problem. During the final stage of life, the benzodiazepines are often very effective, especially when used together with opiates, in controlling terminal anxiety and air hunger. Earlier in the disease, a low-dose, short-acting benzodiazepine is often tolerated and can be used with careful monitoring for signs of carbon dioxide retention (eg, headache, somnolence, and confusion).

Pain

Pain is reported by about half of patients with ALS. Pain is not directly caused by ALS, but rather the symptom results from immobility and weakness. Physical therapy and optimal seating and bed arrangements can often prevent or limit pain, but pharmacologic intervention is often necessary. The first line of pharmacologic treatment is acetaminophen because it lacks major side effects; nonsteroidal anti-inflammatory drugs are also useful. For localized superficial pain, lidocaine in patches or cream can be used. Similar to the before-mentioned benzodiazepines, opiates act as respiratory depressants, and this complicates their use in the respiratory challenged ALS population in a similar way.

Spasticity

Spasticity is a significant problem for many patients with ALS with upper motor neuron dominant disease. Although physical therapy is the first line of therapy, medications are often useful. Baclofen and other muscle relaxants often provide adequate relief without problematic sedation or other side effects. Dosing before bedtime or divided up to 4 times per day can be tried depending on when the symptom is most troubling. All types of pharmacologic management for spasticity result in functional muscle weakness, so reduced spasticity will need to be balanced against the strength loss to achieve optimal function for the patient. When oral muscle relaxants cause too much sedation, then intrathecal baclofen delivered by an implantable pump can be very useful. Patients selected for the procedure should be robust enough to tolerate surgery without a protracted recovery and have a life expectancy in which they would have a chance of benefiting from the procedure. Botulinum toxin can be used with great effect providing targeted and fairly local effect on the muscles selected. Because botulinum toxin's mechanism of action is to functionally denervate the target muscle, significant consideration has to be taken into the functional consequence of weakening the spastic muscle. There is the potential for the disease process to advance during the time the muscle is functionally denervated, which will limit the muscle's ability to recover from the botulinum injections.

Muscle cramps

Muscle cramps are a common symptom in ALS, affecting 62% of patients.[39] Nonpharmacologic measures, such as stretching, can often alleviate these symptoms. Quinine was previously the most used medication for treatment of muscle cramps. Quinine is deemed effective by both meta-analyses and by ALS clinicians, and it remains the favored agent outside of the United States.[39,40] The FDA and Health Canada have advised against the use of quinine for muscle cramps because of very rare fatal hematological side effects attributed to quinine. Quinine is still marketed in the United States, making off-label use against muscle cramps possible, but this is contrary to the specific recommendation of the FDA.[40,41] Other medications that can be used include mexiletine, baclofen, and gabapentin.

Fasciculations

Fasciculations are a very treatment-resistant symptom, which often spontaneously diminishes over time. No medications have been proven to reduce the symptom nor are any medications supported by anecdotal evidence.

Sialorrhea

Drooling and the experience of sialorrhea are the result of poor swallowing function in ALS. Saliva production is not increased because of ALS, but reducing saliva production is the most effective way of reducing these symptoms. Nonpharmacologic measures can include napkins, oral suction machines, and addressing any dental problems. Anticholinergic medications effectively reduce saliva production and glycopyrrolate can be very effective. Other anticholinergics commonly used are atropine drops and scopolamine patches. Anticholinergic medications can cause a dry mouth, constipation, confusion, and worsening of balance, but if one of these side effects limits use, then other options are available. Botulinum toxin directed at the salivary glands is often used, but radiation and even surgery can be used to reduce secretions.

Laryngospasms

Laryngospasm occurs owing to airway spasticity in ALS. It can be caused by dysphagia, but often the cause is gastroesophageal reflux from the stomach. The airway cramp is often brief, but the symptom can be terrifying. If a patient loses consciousness from laryngospasm obstructing the airway, the spasm is relieved. Informing patients that the spasm will not be fatal can offer some reassurance for the patient. Preventive treatment with proton pump inhibitors is normally effective and more practical than attempts of abortive treatment with nitroglycerin or benzodiazepines. The brief duration of attacks and potential choking hazard of oral administration of medications during an attack makes the abortive options less attractive.

Secretion management

Respiratory secretions can be troubling to patients with ALS with reduced pharyngeal function and weak cough. Nonpharmacologic interventions include in/exsufflators and chest percussion. It is important to determine whether the problem is the thickness of the secretions or if the secretions are excessive, because the treatments differ. Anticholinergic medications effectively reduce secretion production and glycopyrrolate can also be very effective. The problem with reducing secretions is that any remaining secretion will be thicker and this can be more troubling for some patients. To liquefy secretions, improved hydration is often a useful first step. Medications that can have an effect on thinning secretions are guaifenesin, acetylcysteine nebulization, and beta-blockers.

Urinary urgency

Urinary urgency is yet another common problem in ALS. Anticholinergics are again useful. Tolterodine has a more bladder-specific effect and thus may be the best choice, but other anticholinergic agents are also useful. Botulinum toxin injections into the bladder detrusor muscle are another option.

In summary, these medications can help alleviate many of the difficult symptoms of ALS, and pharmacologic management of ALS can significantly improve the quality of life for the person suffering from the disease. The role of symptom management in ALS can be expected to increase as we achieve longer survival until there is a treatment that can reverse the condition. A summary of pharmacologic management options for managing ALS is in **Table 1**.

PHARMACOLOGIC MANAGEMENT OF THE IDIOPATHIC INFLAMMATORY MYOPATHIES

The common idiopathic inflammatory myopathies (IIM) include polymyositis (PM), dermatomyositis (DM), autoimmune necrotizing myopathy (ANM), and inclusion body myositis (IBM). There are no evidence-based medications approved by the FDA for the treatment of myositis, and there is little good-quality evidence on which to base treatment recommendations. Also affecting any review of the IIM is that there is no classification of the IIM disorders that is generally agreed on.[42] The Bohan and Peter criteria are obsolete, only defining PM and DM.[43,44] The 3 IIM (PM, DM, and ANM) that

Table 1
Medications commonly used to manage symptoms in ALS

Target	Medication	Typical Dose	Comment
ALS	Riluzole	50 mg BID	Periodic liver function testing
PBA	Dextromethorphan/quinidine	20/10 mg BID	
	Fluoxetine (or other SSRI)[a]	20–80 mg QD	
	Amitriptyline (or other TCA)[a]	10–75 mg BID	
Fatigue	Modafinil[a]	100–200 mg QAM	
	Fluoxetine (or other activating SSRI)[a]	20–80 mg QD	
Spasticity	Baclofen	10–80 mg divided over 24 h	
Muscle cramps	Quinine[a]	324 mg QHS	
	Mexiletine[a]	200 mg BID	
	Gabapentin[a]	1200 mg TID	
Sialorrhea	Glycopyrrolate[a]	1–2 mg QD to QID	
	Scopolamine patch[a]	1.5 mg Q 3 d	
	Atropine 1% solution[a]	1–4 gtt Q 2 h PRN	
Laryngospasm	Omeprazole[a]	20 mg QD	
Respiratory secretions	Glucopyrrolate[a]	1–2 mg QD to QID	
	Guaifenesin	200–400 mg Q 4 h	
	Acetylcysteine 20%	3–5 mL TID PRN	

Abbreviations: ALS, amyotrophic lateral sclerosis; BID, twice a day; gtt, drops; PBA, pseudobulbar affect; PRN, as needed; QAM, every morning; QD, every day; QHS, each bedtime; QID, 4 times daily; SSRI, selective serotonin reuptake inhibitor; TCA, tricyclic antidepressant; TID, 3 times a day.
[a] Off-label use.

are generally accepted to be immune mediated, do have the same basic treatments and will be discussed together as a group. Inclusion body myositis for which the issue of whether the disease is primarily immune mediated remains contentious and is discussed separately.

Pharmacologic Management of Autoimmune Inflammatory Myopathies

Clinically PM, DM, and ANM present with proximal muscle weakness often subacutely with markedly (>5× upper limit of normal) elevated creatine kinase (CK) values. In clinical care, the diagnoses are made by combining the clinical features with histologic findings. Polymyositis is a disease histologically characterized by endomysial inflammation. In dermatomyositis, the inflammation tends to be perifascicular and perivascular within the muscle and also involves the dermis. The increasingly used label of autoimmune necrotizing myopathy is an immune myopathy that lacks the mononuclear cellular infiltrates that are characteristic of the other inflammatory myopathies. The disorder responds to immunosuppressant treatments much like PM and DM, and practically it appears in many ways similar to these IIM. ANM is often caused by antibodies directed against 3-hydroxy-3-methyl-glutaryl-CoA reductase (HMG-CR), an enzyme that is upregulated by statin treatment; however, antibodies against SRP and paraneoplastic mechanisms also cause the same clinicopathologic appearance. Statin medications should be discontinued in ANM and are relatively contraindicated in the other IIM.

Corticosteroids

Corticosteroids, such as prednisone, are the mainstay of immunosuppression for PM, DM, and ANM. Prednisone acts quickly and strength often improves within weeks. Full recovery is generally achieved in the first 6 months. Corticosteroids also have an almost immediate effect on lowering creatine kinase (CK) values.[45] Different prednisone dosing regimens are used. The most common regimens range from 0.5 to 1.5 mg/kg per day. If the treatment is successful and strength is improving to near normal strength, then the corticosteroid should be tapered and eventually discontinued if no disease recurrence is seen. Gradually reducing the dose in half by moving from daily dosing to every other day is a common strategy. If this is successful without recurrence of weakness, then doses can be spaced even further or the dose lowered. If symptoms recur, the dose needs to be increased back to the lowest effective dose. To reduce long-term corticosteroid side effects, either a corticosteroid dose modification or reduction is normally warranted. Pulsed corticosteroids or pulsed dosing regimen can achieve disease control with fewer side effects.[46] Often a steroid-sparing agent is more effective in reducing long-term side effects of corticosteroids. Corticosteroid treatment should be preceded by an evaluation of active and chronic infections that could be worsened by immunosuppression. With long-term treatment, periodic monitoring of blood counts, blood sugar, bone density, weight, hyperlipidemia, and hypertension is advisable.

Steroid-sparing immunosuppression

For most patients, a second-line steroid-sparing immunosuppressant is the best treatment option. Steroid-sparing immunosuppressants can be needed because of steroid treatment failure or need for long-term treatment. There is not a strong evidence base for the use of steroid-sparing immunosuppressants, but empirically many have been used extensively. The most commonly used agent is methotrexate. Methotrexate is usually dosed at 15 to 25 mg per week when taken orally. Folate supplementation should be used together with methotrexate, as it reduces the hematological side effects from the medication. Methotrexate can cause pulmonary fibrosis and, therefore, it is best not used in the IIM patients who have concomitant interstitial lung disease. Periodic blood count and liver function monitoring should be done. Other oral immunosuppressant alternatives include azathioprine and mycophenolate mofetil.[47–49] Intravenous immunoglobulin (IVIG) can also be used and has a role in treating acute or recalcitrant disease.[50] Rituximab infusions have also been used with good effect in some cases.[51] Polymyositis, DM, and ANM conditions can all occur secondary to a neoplastic process. If they are associated with a paraneoplastic process, the primary target for treatment should be the underlying malignancy.

Pharmacologic Management of Inclusion Body Myositis

Inclusion body myositis (IBM) is believed to be a primary inflammatory myopathy by some authorities,[52] but others regard it as a myodegenerative condition.[53] Clinically, it is usually distinguishable from the other IIM because of its slower rate of progression and because of its often distal and asymmetrical distribution of weakness. Although there are several case reports describing cases responding to immunosuppression, most patients are not helped by any currently available agents.[54] Chronic immunosuppression is associated with significant negative health effects and patients with IBM on immunosuppressants may do worse over time compared with untreated patients.[55] However, a trial of corticosteroids (or other immunosuppressants) can still be considered in IBM because a small minority of patients do respond to such treatment, particularly if the IBM diagnosis is uncertain.

PHARMACOLOGIC MANAGEMENT OF NEUROMUSCULAR JUNCTION DISORDERS

The neuromuscular junction (NMJ) is the target of a number of diseases. The most common, myasthenia gravis (MG) and Lambert Eaton myasthenic syndrome (LEMS), are autoimmune in origin, but genetically determined disorders or so-called congenital myasthenic syndromes (CMS) also occur. The treatment of each of these diseases has been enhanced by the accumulating knowledge of the pathogenic mechanisms at work to reduce transmission across this cholinergic (nicotinic) synapse.

Neuromuscular Junction Physiology

The NMJ consists of the specialized nerve terminal of the motor neuron axon separated by a narrow synaptic cleft from the specialized muscle endplate (EP).[56] Motor nerve action potentials depolarize the nerve terminal activating the voltage-gated calcium channels (VGCCs) leading to Ca2+ ion influx. The influx of Ca2+ leads to release of the neurotransmitter acetylcholine (ACh) into the synaptic cleft. ACh diffuses across the cleft to the EP and binds to the densely packed acetylcholine receptors (AChRs) on the peaks of the highly folded EP membrane. ACh binding results in opening of the AChR cation pore. The flux of sodium and potassium depolarizes the membrane and initiates a muscle action potential leading to muscle contraction. ACh then further diffuses into the valleys of the folds, where acetylcholine esterase (AChE) hydrolyzes (inactivates) the neurotransmitter.

Neuromuscular Junction Pathophysiology

In MG, autoantibodies (autoAb) target the AChR, reducing the effective postsynaptic EP concentration of AChRs via 3 mechanisms: increased turnover of AChRs, complement-mediated EP membrane destruction, and pharmacologic blockade of AChR function.[57] Reduced AChR lowers the probability of the initiation of a resultant muscle action potential. In contrast, the autoAb target in LEMS is the presynaptic nerve terminal VGCCs leading to reduced neurotransmitter (ACh) release and resulting in reduced likelihood of initiation of a muscle action potential.[58] Because the VGCCs are much less concentrated, the autoAbs appear to effect VGCC concentration only by direct blockade and increased turnover. For the multitude of forms of CMS, any protein involved in synaptic transmission including AChE is a potential site of disease-inducing mutations.

Symptomatic Pharmacologic Management of MG

A major contribution to the improved prognosis of MG has derived from symptomatic treatment of the disease including general medical advances in critical care medicine.[59] In most cases, the first-line treatment is the symptomatic use of AChE inhibitors (eg, pyridostigmine), which increases the lifetime of ACh at the EP driving by mass action the activation of the remaining AChRs. The use of such agents can be considered symptomatic treatment in the sense that they do not affect the primary pathogenic process: Ab-induced reduction in AChR concentration. AChE inhibitors have an excellent safety profile and in mild cases may adequately control symptoms. In more severe cases, AChE inhibitors may initially control symptoms; however, with time, the effect wanes presumably because the ongoing loss of EP AChRs outstrips the ability AChE inhibitors to maximally activate the remaining AChRs.

Immune-directed Pharmacologic Management of MG

The next step in treatment is targeted at the abnormal immune system in these patients.[59] These modalities have significant side effects and risks but have led to marked improvements in the care of patients with MG. At every step of the way, risks have to be weighed against benefits. These treatments are generally divided according to their speed of action and duration of action into *short*-acting agents and *long*-acting agents.

Short-acting treatments

The short-acting modalities comprise plasma exchange (PE) and IVIG. PE has been used for many years in MG for a rapid effect, especially in patients with myasthenic crisis (respiratory failure on the basis of decreased ventilation or decreased airway protection) or impending myasthenic crisis. Hence, PE was considered the first-line modality in this category[60]; however, evidence-based analyses including a head-to-head randomized controlled clinical trial have determined that IVIG is equally effective.[61,62] Moreover, the head-to-head clinical trial determined that the rate of serious adverse events from PE is significantly greater than for IVIG, primarily as a result of the large-bore intravenous catheter required for PE. Other uses of the short-acting agents are the rapid treatment of exacerbations that occur as a result of tapering immunosuppressive agents, infection, or surgery. PE and IVIG are also used for induction of rapid improvement while waiting for the effect of the long-acting agents (see the next section) to begin. Occasionally in steroid-dependent patients (see later in this article), PE and IVIG can help lower the steroid dose.

Long-acting treatments

The long-acting agents represent the more definitive treatment of the disease. They are slow to act but their effects are long-lived. The first-line modalities include thymectomy (in patients in the appropriate age group), which has the advantage in general of the absence of side effects after the perioperative period. The absence of randomized controlled clinical trials demonstrating the efficacy of thymectomy has led to the initiation of such a trial, which has not yet been completed.[63] It is of note that except for the azathioprine as a steroid-sparing agent (see later in this article),[64] none of the modalities in this category have class I evidence of efficacy.

The mainstay of MG pharmacologic management is adrenocortical steroids.[59] High-dose treatment results in remission of MG in about 80% of patients. The effect usually begins about 4 to 8 weeks after initiating treatment. In some patients, a temporary worsening of symptoms occurs from 10 to 14 days after beginning treatment. The frequency of this side effect can be reduced by gradual increases in the steroid dosage or by a course of IVIG at the time of initiation of steroid treatment. Because of the high risk/benefit ratio of steroids, the dose is slowly tapered to the minimal effective dose once remission is established. In a small number of patients, the MG flairs after only minimal dose reduction, so-called steroid dependence.

Cytotoxic immunosuppressants, including azathioprine, mycophenolate mofetil, cyclosporine, cyclophosphamide and, perhaps, rituximab represent the second line of treatment. Although many of these agents have a better safety profile than steroids, they all appear to be less effective in remission induction, and many of them require months of treatment before any effect is seen. They are most effective as steroid-sparing agents, permitting dose reductions in steroid-dependent patients.

Pharmacologic Management of LEMS

LEMS, like MG, is an autoimmune disorder. Symptomatic treatment aimed at either increasing the activity of the VGCC or inhibiting AChE activity is generally effective. Immune-directed treatment is often unnecessary except in refractory cases.

Symptomatic treatment of LEMS

Symptomatic treatment either increases the activity of the VGCC or inhibits the activity of AChE. The amount of ACh bound is effectively raised to what is a normal concentration of AChR. Significant improvement in strength is achieved by 3,4-diaminopyridine (DAP), an experimental potassium channel blocker, currently only available on a compassionate use basis.[65] This agent blocks the nerve terminal rectifying potassium channel that is active in the repolarization portion of the nerve action potential. The blockade results in lengthening the duration of the action potential so that the nerve terminal remains depolarized for a longer time leading to a longer period of activation of the remaining VGCCs. The increase in Ca2+ ion flux appears to be sufficient to return ACh release to near normal levels.

Immune-directed treatment of LEMS

It appears that most patients receive sufficient benefit from DAP plus or minus AChE inhibitors to render immune-directed treatment unnecessary. If needed, these treatments include those described previously for MG except for thymectomy, which is not effective in LEMS. For the 50% of patients in which LEMS is a paraneoplastic syndrome resulting from tumor immunity directed against the VGCC-expressing small cell lung carcinoma, excision of the tumor can be effective treatment for LEMS.[66]

Pharmacologic Management of CMSs

Because each form of CMS results from mutations in single members of the various proteins active in neuromuscular transmission, some located presynaptically, some in the synaptic cleft and some in the EP, treatment must be individualized. Two of the more common forms are slow-channel congenital myasthenic syndrome (SCCMS) and AChE deficiency.[67]

Treatment of SCCMS

For SCCMS, the mutation is in the ion pore of the EP AChR and results in prolonged opening of the pore after ACh binding to the AChR. This causes prolonged muscle depolarization, such that the EP remains unresponsive to ACh for an extended period of time, actually blocking NMJ transmission (depolarization block). Over time, the prolonged openings also result in the cytotoxic effects of Ca2+ overload in the muscle EP region. Treatment involves paradoxically blocking the open AChR ion pore with agents such as quinidine.

Treatment of AChE deficiency

In the AChE deficiency form of CMS, exposure of AChR to excess ACh concentrations results in a combination of depolarization block and desensitization of the AChR molecules making them unresponsive for extended periods of time. This disorder is difficult to treat but occasionally patients respond to adrenergic agonists by a mechanism yet to be understood.

PHARMACOLOGIC MANAGEMENT OF MYOTONIA

Myotonia is the disturbance of muscle relaxation experienced by muscle stiffness. Several neuromuscular disorders have myotonia as a symptom. Myotonia is often not as disabling as the underlying weakness but can cause significant discomfort and decrease in function. Myotonia is most commonly seen in the myotonic dystrophies, myotonic dystrophy type I (DM1), and myotonic dystrophy type 2 (DM2). The chloride channelopathies, Thomsen myotonia congenita (autosomal dominant) and Becker myotonia congenita (autosomal recessive), both have symptoms of myotonia.

Paramyotonia congenita is a sodium channel myotonia. Myotonia fluctuans and myotonia permanens are both potassium-aggravated myotonias.[68] Intramuscular fluoxetine reduces electrophysiological myotonia in DM1 but is not a practical treatment option.[69] Mexiletine and tocainide are the most effective antimyotonia treatments but tocainide's potential for bone marrow suppression precludes its long-term use.[70,71] The dosing range for mexiletine is usually 150 to 200 mg 3 times daily. Electrocardiogram parameters should be monitored owing to the risk of arrhythmias.[68,70] Other sodium channel blockers, such as procainamide, phenytoin, disopyramide, and carbamazepine, have also been used to treat myotonia.[68,71,72] In myotonic dystrophies, careful monitoring of muscle strength needs to be implemented if sodium channel blocker therapy is initiated, as sodium channel blockers can also worsen weakness.[68,72] Similar to the myotonic dystrophies, mexiletine is the first-line therapy for the myotonia congenitas and the most effective. Because the myotonia congenitas suffer from myotonia more than weakness, medications are often used. Carbamazepine and phenytoin are also often used. Rarely are medications needed for symptom control in Thomsen myotonia congenita.[68,72] Dietary restriction of potassium is useful in the management of the potassium aggravated myotonias. This class of myotonias also responds well to acetazolamide; however, mexiletine is still considered a first-line therapy.

PHARMACOLOGIC MANAGEMENT OF SELECT PEDIATRIC NEUROMUSCULAR DISORDERS

Despite the accumulating knowledge of the genetics and pathophysiology of hereditary pediatric neuromuscular disorders, no cure has been discovered and only limited pharmacologic treatments are available. The rate of new promising therapeutics coming to the clinical trial phase is encouraging.

Pharmacologic Management of Duchenne Muscular Dystrophy

Duchenne muscular dystrophy (DMD) is caused by mutations in the dystrophin gene, which results in the absence of or defective dystrophin protein. The current standard of care treatment for DMD is corticosteroids.[73] Corticosteroids have prolonged ambulation and decreased the incidence of scoliosis in boys with DMD. There are 3 newer pharmaceutical therapies emerging for the treatment of DMD: mutation-specific exon skipping, the suppression of premature stop codons otherwise known as nonsense mutations, and utrophin upregulation. Exon skipping is an RNA approach that relies on synthesized antisense oligonucleotides to alter splicing. Nonsense mutation suppression promotes read-through of premature stop codons by interfering with the ability of the ribosome to recognize the stop codons. Utrophin upregulation attempts to replace the missing or dysfunctional dystrophin with utrophin, which is similar in structure.[74]

Corticosteroids

Standardized care recommendations for DMD have been published. The recommendations emphasized the importance of corticosteroids in the treatment of DMD. The current recommendations are to initiate daily treatment prednisone at 0.75 mg/kg/d or deflazacort at 0.9 mg/kg/d when function plateaus or starts to decline. Alternative regimens, such as alternate day, high-dose weekend, and 10 days on 10 days off, have also been used. The minimum effective dose for prednisone is thought to be 0.3 mg/kg/d. The maximum recommended dose for prednisone is 30 to 40 mg/d or 36 to 39 mg/d for deflazacort. Aggressive intervention to manage the side effects of the corticosteroids is recommended to prolong the duration of therapy as long as possible or tolerated.[73]

Antisense oligonucleotides

The dystrophin gene is the largest gene in the body, consisting of 79 exons. In most cases of DMD, exons are deleted, which prevents the rest of the remaining exons from being read, resulting in a nonfunctional dystrophin protein. By skipping additional exons, the reading frame can be restored, enabling functional dystrophin protein production. Mutation-specific exon skipping is achieved through the use of antisense oligonucleotides. Antisense oligonucleotides pair with pre-mRNA or mRNA modulating splicing or transcription. The main application of antisense oligonucleotides in DMD has been to restore the open reading frame in out-of-frame deletions. Restoring the open reading in DMD may modify the phenotype to the allelic but less-affected condition of Becker muscular dystrophy.[75] Preliminary studies of exon 51 skipping are promising.[76,77] A Phase III systemic clinical trial for antisense oligonucleotides exon 51 skipping is currently under way. The concomitant use of prednisone and antisense oligonucleotides resulted in higher dystrophin expression in the mdx mouse in comparison with those treated with antisense oligonucleotides alone. This suggests that current standard of care therapy for DMD may augment antisense oligonucleotide efficacy and is not a barrier to clinical trial participation.[78] The specificity of antisense treatment may preclude is application in general medical care of NMD owing to the high cost of research, development, and production. If antisense therapy proves affective, an antisense oligonucleotide skipping exons 45 to 55 would be an applicable treatment for up to 63% of boys with DMD.[79,80]

Nonsense mutation suppression

Around 10% to 15% of boys with DMD have a nonsense mutation resulting in a premature stopped codon. Ataluren or PTC124 is a compound that was identified by high-throughput screening to bind to the 60S ribosomal subunit and read-through premature stop codons with no evidence of ribosomal read-through of normal stop codons (**Fig. 1**). Ataluren has been shown to increase dystrophin production in the mdx mouse by 20% to 25% in comparison with the wild-type mouse. Although the primary outcome measurement was not reached in the Phase IIb study, ongoing efforts to demonstrate its clinical efficacy in DMD are under way.[75,81,82]

Utrophin upregulation

Utrophin is a chromosome 6 gene that is 80% identical in sequence to dystrophin. Utrophin is expressed in muscles during embryonic development. In adult myofibers, it is only expressed in neuromuscular junctions and at the myotendinous junctions. The translational inhibition of utrophin in adult myofibers is mediated by microRNA (miRNA). Blocking the function of the miRNA may derepress the translation of utrophin.[83] A threefold to fourfold increase in expression of utrophin in muscle fibers of the mdx mouse almost corrected the dystrophic phenotype.[81] Utrophin upregulation has the advantage in that it would be applicable in all patients with DMD or Becker muscular dystrophy and may be beneficial in muscular dystrophies.[79] A phase I clinical trial attempting to upregulate utrophin expression failed to do show any physiologic effect owing to the compounds pharmokinetics.[81]

Myostatin inhibition

Myostatin is a growth factor-β that regulates muscle size. In animals with myostatin gene knockout, significant muscle hypertrophy is observed. Modulation of the myostatin pathway can be achieved through the decrease in production of the myostatin

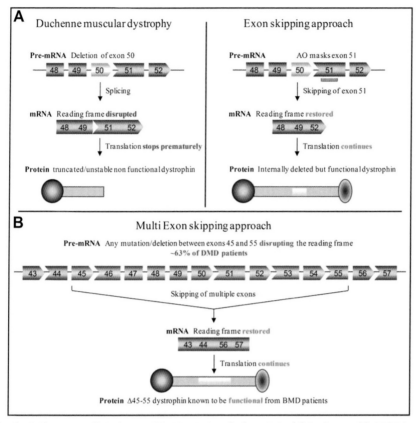

Fig. 1. Antisense-mediated exon skipping rationale for DMD. (*A*) Patients with DMD have mutations that disrupt the open reading frame of the dystrophin pre-mRNA. In this example, exon 50 is deleted, creating an out-of-frame mRNA and leading to the synthesis of a truncated nonfunctional or unstable dystrophin (*left panel*). An antisense oligonucleotide directed against exon 51 can induce effective skipping of exon 51 and restore the open reading frame, therefore generating an internally deleted but partly functional dystrophin (*right panel*). (*B*) Multiple exon-skipping rationale for DMD. The optimal skipping of exons 45 to 55 leading to the del45–55 artificial dystrophin could transform the DMD phenotype into the asymptomatic or mild BMD phenotype. This multiple exon skipping could theoretically rescue up to 63% of patients with DMD with a deletion. (*From* Goyenvalle A, Seto JT, Davies KE, et al. Therapeutic approaches to muscular dystrophy [review]. Hum Mol Genet 2011;20(R1):R69–78; with permission.)

peptide or modulating the binding to its receptor, the activin type-II receptor. Blockade of the activin IIB receptor led to increased muscle mass and muscle force generation in the mdx mouse.[84] A clinical trial using an antibody against myostatin (MYO-029) was undertaken, which failed to demonstrate any significant improvements in muscle strength.[85] Increasing dystrophin or utrophin production could be coupled with myostatin inhibition to collectively improve the phenotype in DMD.[86] Additionally, myostatin inhibition may be beneficial in other muscular dystrophies and myopathies.

Idebenone
Idebenone is a synthetic analog of coenzyme Q10 with strong antioxidant activities, which in addition improves mitochondrial respiratory chain function and cellular

energy production. A phase IIa double-blind randomized placebo-controlled clinical trial was conducted to investigate the tolerability and efficacy of idebenone therapy in children with DMD. There was a significant treatment effect favoring idebenone on peak expiratory flow, both in absolute value and %predicted.[87] A phase III study evaluating muscle strength in under way.

Pharmacologic Management of Spinal Muscular Atrophy

Antisense oligonucleotide strategies have also been evaluated in the treatment of spinal muscular atrophy (SMA). SMA is caused by loss of function mutations in the survival motor neuron 1 (SMN1) gene. There is no proven efficacious medication treatment for SMA type I, II, or III.[88,89] The disease severity is primarily determined by the copy number of survival motor neuron 2 (SMN2) gene, which produces a protein with similar function to the SMN1 gene but in much lower quantities.[90] Single nucleotide polymorphisms (SNPs) in exon 7 of SMN2 cause a high proportion of exon 7 skipping during pre-mRNA splicing leading to an unstable truncated SMN protein. As a result, small levels of functional SMN protein are produced by the SMN2 gene. Restoring the splicing to achieve exon 7 inclusion has the potential to produce sufficient quantities of functional protein to compensate for the deficit of SMN1 protein.[75,91] The systemic delivery of antisense oligonucleotides significantly improves the phenotype of the mouse model of SMA.[91] A phase I clinical study is currently under way exploring antisense oligonucleotides as a therapeutic option for patients with SMA. There is also a phase I clinical trial under way investigating a novel compound that has shown to increase SMN2 protein production in mice and cell culture.[92]

SUMMARY

The growing knowledge of neuromuscular disorders presents new opportunities and strategies for pharmacologic interventions. Although they are no cures, there are many interventions that can improve the natural history of the various conditions. Symptomatic treatments improve the function and increase the quality of life for those suffering from neuromuscular disorders. The future remains optimistic for significant pharmacologic interventions and possibly cures.

REFERENCES

1. Pompe JC. Over idioptische hypertrophie van het hart. Ned Tidschr Geneeskd 1932;76:304–11.
2. Kishnani PS, Howell RR. Pompe disease in infants and children. J Pediatr 2004; 144:S35–43.
3. Cori GT. Biochemical aspects of glycogen deposition disease. Mod Probl Paediatr 1957;3:344–58.
4. Hers HG. Alpha-glucosidase deficiency in generalized glycogen-storage disease (Pompe's disease). Biochem J 1963;86:11–6.
5. de Duve C, Pressman B, Gianetto T, et al. Tissue fractionation studies. Biochem J 1955;60:604–17.
6. Engel AG, Seybold ME, Lambert EH, et al. Acid maltase deficiency: comparison of infantile, childhood, and adult types. Neurology 1970;20:382.
7. American Association of Neuromuscular & Electrodiagnostic Medicine. Diagnostic criteria for late-onset (childhood and adult) Pompe disease. Muscle Nerve 2009;40:149–60.
8. Raben N, Roberts A, Plotz PH. Role of autophagy in the pathogenesis of Pompe disease. Acta Myol 2007;26:45–8.

9. Reuser AJ, Drost MR. Lysosomal dysfunction, cellular pathology and clinical symptoms: basic principles. Acta Paediatr Suppl 2006;95:77–82.

10. Hirschhorn R, Reuser AJ. Glycogen storage disease type II: acid a-glucosidase (acid maltase) deficiency. Scriver's MMBID website. Available at: http://www.ommbid.com//OMMBID/the_online_metabolic_and_molecular_bases_of_inherited_disease/b/abstract/part16/ch135. Accessed September 9, 2012.

11. Kishnani PS, Steiner RD, Bali D, et al. Pompe disease diagnosis and management guideline. Genet Med 2006;8:267–88.

12. Kishnani PS, Hwu WL, Mandel H, et al. A retrospective, multinational, multicenter study on the natural history of infantile-onset Pompe disease. J Pediatr 2006;148: 671–6.

13. de Barsy T, Jacquemin P, Van Hoof F, et al. Enzyme replacement in Pompe disease: an attempt with purified human acid alpha-glucosidase. Birth Defects Orig Artic Ser 1973;9:184–90.

14. Van den Hout JM, Kamphoven JH, Winkel LP, et al. Long-term intravenous treatment of Pompe disease with recombinant human alpha-glucosidase from milk. Pediatrics 2004;113:e448–57.

15. Honig J, Martiniuk F, D'Eustachio P, et al. Confirmation of the regional localization of the genes for human acid alpha-glucosidase (GAA) and adenosine deaminase (ADA) by somatic cell hybridization. Ann Hum Genet 1984;48:49–56.

16. MYOZYME [package insert]. Cambridge (MA): Genzyme Corporation; 2010.

17. Kishnani PS, Nicolino M, Voit T, et al. Chinese hamster ovary cell-derived recombinant human acid alpha-glucosidase in infantile-onset Pompe disease. J Pediatr 2006;149:89–97.

18. van der Ploeg AT, Clemens P, Corzo D, et al. A randomized study of alglucosidase alfa in late-onset Pompe's disease. N Engl J Med 2010;362:1396–406.

19. LUMIZYME [package insert]. Cambridge (MA): Genzyme Corporation; 2010.

20. Cupler EJ, Berger KI, Leshner RT, et al. Consensus Committee on Late-onset Pompe Disease. Consensus treatment recommendations for late-onset Pompe disease. Muscle Nerve 2012;45(3):319–33.

21. Barba-Romero MA, Barrot E, Bautista-Lorite J, et al. Clinical guidelines for late-onset Pompe disease. Rev Neurol 2012;54(8):497–507.

22. Genzyme. Lumizyme ACE program. Available at: http://www.lumizyme.com/ace/. Accessed July 13, 2012.

23. Rothstein JD. Therapeutic horizons for amyotrophic lateral sclerosis. Curr Opin Neurobiol 1996;6:679–87.

24. Cheah BC, Vucic S, Krishnan AV, et al. Riluzole, neuroprotection and amyotrophic lateral sclerosis. Curr Med Chem 2010;17:1942–99.

25. Gurney ME, Fleck TJ, Himes CS, et al. Riluzole preserves motor function in a transgenic model of familial amyotrophic lateral sclerosis. Neurology 1998;50:62–6.

26. Bensimon G, Lacomblez L, Meininger V. A controlled trial of riluzole in amyotrophic lateral sclerosis. ALS/Riluzole Study Group. N Engl J Med 1994;330:585–91.

27. Lacomblez L, Bensimon G, Leigh PN, et al. Dose-ranging study of riluzole in amyotrophic lateral sclerosis. Amyotrophic Lateral Sclerosis/Riluzole Study Group II. Lancet 1996;347:1425–31.

28. Bensimon G, Lacomblez L, Delumeau JC, et al. A study of riluzole in the treatment of advanced stage or elderly patients with amyotrophic lateral sclerosis. J Neurol 2002;249:609–15.

29. Bradley WG, Anderson F, Gowda N, et al. Changes in the management of ALS since the publication of the AAN ALS practice parameter 1999. Amyotroph Lateral Scler Other Motor Neuron Disord 2004;5:240–4.

30. Miller RG, Mitchell JD, Moore DH. Riluzole for amyotrophic lateral sclerosis (ALS)/ motor neuron disease (MND). Cochrane Database Syst Rev 2012;(3):CD001447.
31. Rothstein JD, Patel S, Regan MR, et al. Beta-lactam antibiotics offer neuroprotection by increasing glutamate transporter expression. Nature 2005;433:73–7.
32. Cudkowicz M, Bozik ME, Ingersoll EW, et al. The effects of dexpramipexole (KNS-760704) in individuals with amyotrophic lateral sclerosis. Nat Med 2011;17: 1652–6.
33. Gallagher JP. Pathologic laughter and crying in ALS: a search for their origin. Acta Neurol Scand 1989;80:114–7.
34. Cummings JL, Arciniegas DB, Brooks BR, et al. Defining and diagnosing involuntary emotional expression disorder. CNS Spectr 2006;11:1–7.
35. Pioro EP, Brooks BR, Cummings J, et al. Dextromethorphan plus ultra low-dose quinidine reduces pseudobulbar affect. Ann Neurol 2010;68:693–702.
36. Schiffer RB, Herndon RM, Rudick RA. Treatment of pathologic laughing and weeping with amitriptyline. N Engl J Med 1985;312:1480–2.
37. Murphy JM, Henry RG, Langmore S, et al. Continuum of frontal lobe impairment in amyotrophic lateral sclerosis. Arch Neurol 2007;64:530–4.
38. Rabkin JG, Gordon PH, McElhiney M, et al. Modafinil treatment of fatigue in patients with ALS: a placebo-controlled study. Muscle Nerve 2009;39:297–303.
39. Heiman-Patterson T, Rampai N, Branagan TH, et al. The spectrum of patient symptoms in ALS and symptom management. Neurology 2001;56(Supp 3):A199.
40. El-Tawil S, Al Musa T, Valli H, et al. Quinine for muscle cramps. Cochrane Database Syst Rev 2010;(12):CD005044.
41. FDA Drug Safety Communication: New risk management plan and patient Medication Guide for Qualaquin (quinine sulfate). Available at: http://www.fda.gov/ Drugs/DrugSafety/PostmarketDrugSafetyInformationforPatientsandProviders/ucm 218202.htm. Accessed September 9, 2012.
42. Pestronk A. Acquired immune and inflammatory myopathies: pathologic classification. Curr Opin Rheumatol 2011;23:595–604.
43. Bohan A, Peter JB. Polymyositis and dermatomyositis (first of two parts). N Engl J Med 1975;292:344–7.
44. Bohan A, Peter JB. Polymyositis and dermatomyositis (second of two parts). N Engl J Med 1975;292:403–7.
45. Minetto MA, Botter A, Lanfranco F, et al. Muscle fiber conduction slowing and decreased levels of circulating muscle proteins after short-term dexamethasone administration in healthy subjects. J Clin Endocrinol Metab 2010;95:1663–71.
46. Van de Vlekkert J, Hoogendijk JE, de Haan RJ, et al. Oral dexamethasone pulse therapy versus daily prednisolone in sub-acute onset myositis, a randomised clinical trial. Neuromuscul Disord 2010;20:382–9.
47. Bunch TW. Prednisone and azathioprine for polymyositis: long-term followup. Arthritis Rheum 1981;24:45–8.
48. Bunch TW, Worthington JW, Combs JJ, et al. Azathioprine with prednisone for polymyositis. A controlled, clinical trial. Ann Intern Med 1980;92:365–9.
49. Pisoni CN, Cuadrado MJ, Khamashta MA, et al. Mycophenolate mofetil treatment in resistant myositis. Rheumatology (Oxford) 2007;46:516–8.
50. Dalakas MC, Illa I, Dambrosia JM, et al. A controlled trial of high-dose intravenous immune globulin infusions as treatment for dermatomyositis. N Engl J Med 1993; 329:1993–2000.
51. Levine TD. Rituximab in the treatment of dermatomyositis: an open-label pilot study. Arthritis Rheum 2005;52:601–7.
52. Greenberg SA. Inclusion body myositis. Curr Opin Rheumatol 2011;23:574–8.

53. Askanas V, Engel WK, Nogalska A. Inclusion body myositis: a degenerative muscle disease associated with intra-muscle fiber multi-protein aggregates, proteasome inhibition, endoplasmic reticulum stress and decreased lysosomal degradation. Brain Pathol 2009;19:493–506.

54. Chahin N, Engel AG. Correlation of muscle biopsy, clinical course, and outcome in PM and sporadic IBM. Neurology 2008;70:418–24.

55. Benveniste O, Guiguet M, Freebody J, et al. Long-term observational study of sporadic inclusion body myositis. Brain 2011;134:3176–84.

56. Hughes BW, Kusner LL, Kaminski HJ. Molecular architecture of the neuromuscular junction. Muscle Nerve 2006;33(4):445–61.

57. Vincent A. Immunology of disorders of neuromuscular transmission. Acta Neurol Scand, Suppl 2006;183:1–7.

58. Newsom-Davis J. Lambert-Eaton myasthenic syndrome. Rev Neurol (Paris) 2004; 160(2):177–80.

59. Richman DP, Agius MA. Treatment of autoimmune myasthenia gravis. Neurology 2003;61(12):1652–61.

60. Pinching AJ, Peters DK, Davis JN. Plasma exchange in myasthenia gravis. Lancet 1977;1(8008):428–9.

61. Gajdos P, Chevret S, Toyka K. Intravenous immunoglobulin for myasthenia gravis. Cochrane Database Syst Rev 2008;(1):CD002277.

62. Gajdos P, Chevret S, Clair B, et al. Clinical trial of plasma exchange and high-dose intravenous immunoglobulin in myasthenia gravis. Myasthenia Gravis Clinical Study Group. Ann Neurol 1997;41(6):789–96.

63. Gronseth GS, Barohn RJ. Practice parameter: thymectomy for autoimmune myasthenia gravis (an evidence-based review): report of the Quality Standards Subcommittee of the American Academy of Neurology. Neurology 2000;55(1):7–15.

64. Palace J, Newsom-Davis J, Lecky B. A randomized double-blind trial of prednisolone alone or with azathioprine in myasthenia gravis. Myasthenia Gravis Study Group. Neurology 1998;50(6):1778–83.

65. Wirtz PW, Titulaer MJ, Gerven JM, et al. 3,4-diaminopyridine for the treatment of Lambert-Eaton myasthenic syndrome. Expert Rev Clin Immunol 2010;6(6):867–74.

66. Chalk CH, Murray NM, Newsom-Davis J, et al. Response of the Lambert-Eaton myasthenic syndrome to treatment of associated small-cell lung carcinoma. Neurology 1990;40(10):1552–6.

67. Engel AG. Current status of the congenital myasthenic syndromes. Neuromuscul Disord 2012;22(2):99–111.

68. Lehmann-Horn F, Jurkat-Rott K, Rüdel R, et al. Diagnostics and therapy of muscle channelopathies–Guidelines of the Ulm Muscle Centre [review]. Acta Myol 2008; 27:98–113.

69. Chisari C, Licitra R, Pellegrini M, et al. Fluoxetine blocks myotonic runs and reverts abnormal surface electromyogram pattern in patients with myotonic dystrophy type 1. Clin Neuropharmacol 2009;32(6):330–4.

70. Logigian EL, Martens WB, Moxley RT 4th, et al. Mexiletine is an effective antimyotonia treatment in myotonic dystrophy type 1. Neurology 2010;74(18):1441–8.

71. Kwieciński H, Ryniewicz B, Ostrzycki A. Treatment of myotonia with antiarrhythmic drugs. Acta Neurol Scand 1992;86(4):371–5.

72. Kurihara T. New classification and treatment for myotonic disorders [review]. Intern Med 2005;44(10):1027–32.

73. Bushby K, Finkel R, Birnkrant DJ, et al. Diagnosis and management of Duchenne muscular dystrophy, part 1: diagnosis, and pharmacological and psychosocial management [review]. Lancet Neurol 2010;9(1):77–93.

74. Fairclough RJ, Bareja A, Davies KE. Progress in therapy for Duchenne muscular dystrophy [review]. Exp Physiol 2011;96(11):1101–13.

75. Muntoni F, Wood MJ. Targeting RNA to treat neuromuscular disease [review]. Nat Rev Drug Discov 2011;10(8):621–37. http://dx.doi.org/10.1038/nrd3459.

76. Cirak S, Arechavala-Gomeza V, Guglieri M, et al. Exon skipping and dystrophin restoration in patients with Duchenne muscular dystrophy after systemic phosphorodiamidate morpholino oligomer treatment: an open-label, phase 2, dose-escalation study. Lancet 2011;378(9791):595–605.

77. Goemans NM, Tulinius M, van den Akker JT, et al. Systemic administration of PRO051 in Duchenne's muscular dystrophy [Erratum in N Engl J Med 2011;365(14):1361]. N Engl J Med 2011;364(16):1513–22.

78. Verhaart IE, Heemskerk H, Karnaoukh TG, et al. Prednisolone treatment does not interfere with 2'-O-methyl phosphorothioate antisense-mediated exon skipping in Duchenne muscular dystrophy. Hum Gene Ther 2012;23(3):262–73.

79. Goyenvalle A, Seto JT, Davies KE, et al. Therapeutic approaches to muscular dystrophy [review]. Hum Mol Genet 2011;20(R1):R69–78.

80. Béroud C, Tuffery-Giraud S, Matsuo M, et al. Multiexon skipping leading to an artificial DMD protein lacking amino acids from exons 45 through 55 could rescue up to 63% of patients with Duchenne muscular dystrophy. Hum Mutat 2007;28(2):196–202.

81. Pichavant C, Aartsma-Rus A, Clemens PR, et al. Current status of pharmaceutical and genetic therapeutic approaches to treat DMD [review]. Mol Ther 2011;19(5): 830–40.

82. Finkel RS. Read-through strategies for suppression of nonsense mutations in Duchenne/Becker muscular dystrophy: aminoglycosides and ataluren (PTC124) [review]. J Child Neurol 2010;25(9):1158–64.

83. Basu U, Lozynska O, Moorwood C, et al. Translational regulation of utrophin by miRNAs. PLoS One 2011;6(12):e29376.

84. Morine KJ, Bish LT, Selsby JT, et al. Activin IIB receptor blockade attenuates dystrophic pathology in a mouse model of Duchenne muscular dystrophy. Muscle Nerve 2010;42(5):722–30.

85. Wagner KR, Fleckenstein JL, Amato AA, et al. A phase I/II trial of MYO-029 in adult subjects with muscular dystrophy. Ann Neurol 2008;63(5):561–71.

86. Kemaladewi DU, Hoogaars WM, van Heiningen SH, et al. Dual exon skipping in myostatin and dystrophin for Duchenne muscular dystrophy. BMC Med Genomics 2011;4:36.

87. Buyse GM, Goemans N, van den Hauwe M, et al. Idebenone as a novel, therapeutic approach for Duchenne muscular dystrophy: results from a 12 month, double-blind, randomized placebo-controlled trial. Neuromuscul Disord 2011; 21(6):396–405.

88. Wadman RI, Bosboom WM, van der Pol WL, et al. Drug treatment for spinal muscular atrophy type I. Cochrane Database Syst Rev 2012;(4):CD006281.

89. Wadman RI, Bosboom WM, van der Pol WL, et al. Drug treatment for spinal muscular atrophy types II and III. Cochrane Database Syst Rev 2012;(4):CD006282.

90. Rudnik-Schöneborn S, Berg C, Zerres K, et al. Genotype-phenotype studies in infantile spinal muscular atrophy (SMA) type I in Germany: implications for clinical trials and genetic counselling. Clin Genet 2009;76(2):168–78.

91. MacKenzie A. Sense in antisense therapy for spinal muscular atrophy. N Engl J Med 2012;366(8):761–3.

92. Butchbach ME, Singh J, Thorsteinsdóttir M, et al. Effects of 2,4-diaminoquinazoline derivatives on SMN expression and phenotype in a mouse model for spinal muscular atrophy. Hum Mol Genet 2010;19(3):454–67.

Novel Approaches to Corticosteroid Treatment in Duchenne Muscular Dystrophy

Eric P. Hoffman, PhD[a,b,]*, Erica Reeves, PhD[b], Jesse Damsker, PhD[b],
Kanneboyina Nagaraju, DVM, PhD[a,b], John M. McCall, PhD[b],
Edward M. Connor, MD[a,b], Kate Bushby, MD[c]

KEYWORDS

- Duchenne muscular dystrophy • Corticosteroids • Glucocorticoids
- Dissociative steroids

KEY POINTS

- Current standard of care of Duchenne muscular dystrophy (DMD) includes pharmacologic treatment with oral glucocorticoids.
- Gains in strength and slowed progression of disease afforded by glucocorticoids are offset, in part, by the wide range of side effects of drug treatment.
- Dose optimization studies are limited, and new larger clinical studies are needed to best balance efficacy and side effects (therapeutic window), as are studies of glucocorticoid alternatives to prednisone.
- The FOR-DMD trial funded by the National Institutes of Health is under way to compare different dose regimens and types of glucocorticoids (prednisone, deflazacort).
- A novel dissociative steroid, a Δ-9,11 drug, is under clinical development for DMD. This drug promises to broaden the therapeutic window and reduce side-effect profiles.

INTRODUCTION

Duchenne muscular dystrophy (DMD) is an X-linked progressive muscular dystrophy, caused by loss of the dystrophin protein at the myofiber membrane.[1,2] Pharmacologic treatment of DMD patients with glucocorticoids can improve patient strength and prolong ambulation, with concomitant improvements in quality-of-life scales.[3–9] As

[a] Center for Genetic Medicine Research, Children's National Medical Center, 111 Michigan Avenue Northwest, Washington, DC 20010, USA; [b] ReveraGen Biopharma, 9700 Great Seneca Hwy, Rockville, MD 20850 USA; [c] Institute of Human Genetics, International Centre for Life, Central Parkway, Newcastle upon Tyne NE1 3BZ, UK
* Corresponding author. Center for Genetic Medicine Research, Children's National Medical Center, 111 Michigan Avenue Northwest, Washington, DC 20010.
E-mail address: ehoffman@cnmcresearch.org

Phys Med Rehabil Clin N Am 23 (2012) 821–828
http://dx.doi.org/10.1016/j.pmr.2012.08.003
1047-9651/12/$ – see front matter © 2012 Elsevier Inc. All rights reserved.

such, glucocorticoid treatment for DMD is recommended in standard-of-care guide-lines, and as an American Academy of Neurology practice parameter.[10–12] The majority of trials and treatment recommendations have used an oral dose of predni-sone at 0.75 mg/kg/d. However, alternative dosing regimens have been reported as changing the efficacy versus side-effect profiles, including weekend dosing,[13,14] lower doses,[15] and alternative-day doses (10 mg/kg/wk divided over 2 weekend days).[16–18] In each study, a goal was to achieve a better balance of efficacy (increased strength and delay of disease progression) with fewer side effects (bone fragility, weight gain, mood changes).[19–21] It is pertinent to note that muscle weakness and wasting is an acknowledged side effect of chronic glucocorticoid administration in many indica-tions, such as critical care medicine, and is the most common drug-induced form of muscle weakness.[22] Glucocorticoids have a direct molecular effect on myofibers, stimulating the catabolic AKT1/FOXO1 pathway, decreasing protein synthesis and increasing the rate of protein catabolism, resulting in weakness and atrophy.[23] Thus it is likely that DMD patients treated with glucocorticoids show the clinical outcome of increased muscle strength mitigated to some extent by the side effect of muscle catabolism. Clearly any effort to reduce side effects such as weight gain and short stature may also lead to lessening of the side effect of muscle weakness, whereby the balance would then be tipped to greater efficacy.

Fluorinated glucocorticoids, such as dexamethasone, are considerably more potent, with higher affinity to the glucocorticoid receptor (**Fig. 1**). However, these tend to also exacerbate side effects, and are generally avoided in indications of chronic use, such as muscular dystrophy. On the other hand, less potent nonfluori-nated varieties of glucocorticoids have been tried, such as deflazacort. Deflazacort

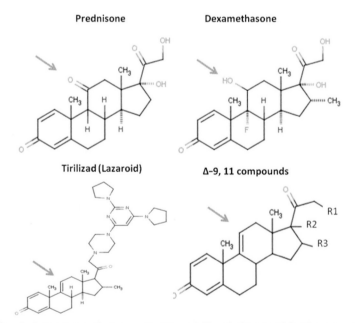

Fig. 1. Chemical structures of glucocorticoids and dissociative steroids. The arrow indicates the position of the key 9,11 alterations distinguishing classic glucocorticoids (prednisone, dexamethasone) from dissociative steroids (Δ-9,11 analogues).

trials in DMD have suggested similar efficacy to that of prednisone (albeit at a higher dose), with an improvement in some side-effect profiles.[3,24–26]

FINDING THE OPTIMUM REGIMEN OF CORTICOSTEROIDS FOR DMD (FOR-DMD) CLINICAL TRIAL

To study the balance of efficacy and side effects, depending on steroid type (prednisone vs deflazcort) and dosing regimen (daily vs 10 days on, 10 days off), the FOR-DMD trial was designed and implemented. FOR-DMD is a multicenter, double-blind, parallel-group, 36- to 60-month study, comparing 3 corticosteroid regimens in wide use in DMD:

- Daily prednisone (0.75 mg/kg/d)
- Intermittent prednisone (0.75 mg/kg/d, 10 days on, 10 days off)
- Daily deflazacort (0.9 mg/kg/d).

The hypothesis being tested is that daily corticosteroids (prednisone or deflazacort) will be of greater benefit than intermittent corticosteroids (prednisone) in terms of function and subject/parent satisfaction. A secondary outcome is to study whether daily deflazacort will be associated with a better side-effect profile than daily prednisone.

The primary outcome variable will be a 3-dimensional (multivariate) outcome consisting of the following 3 components (each averaged over all postbaseline follow-up visits through month 36): (1) time to stand from lying (log-transformed), (2) forced vital capacity, and (3) subject/parent global satisfaction with treatment, as measured by the Treatment Satisfaction Questionnaire for medication.

Secondary outcome variables will include regimen tolerance, adverse event profile, and secondary functional outcomes including the 6-minute walk test, quality of life, and cardiac function. The analyses will be adjusted for covariates, namely country/region, baseline time to stand from lying, baseline forced vital capacity (FVC), and initial weight band. A sample size of 100 subjects per group (300 in total) will provide adequate power to detect differences that are thought to be of minimal clinical significance between any 2 of the 3 treatment groups, assuming a 10% rate of subject withdrawal.

The trial will randomize 300 boys aged 4 to 7 years to 0.75 mg/kg/d prednisone; 0.75 mg/kg/d prednisone for 10 days alternating with 10 days off; or 0.9 mg/kg/d deflazacort. All boys will complete a minimum 3 years (36 months) treatment period. All boys entering the trial will remain on the study drug until the last boy completes the 36 months of study; this may be up to 60 months.

Eligible boys will be those with confirmed DMD (defined as male with clinical signs compatible with DMD and confirmed DMD mutation in the dystrophin gene [out-of-frame deletion or point mutation or duplication] or absent/<3% dystrophin on muscle biopsy); age at least 4 years and under 8 years; ability to rise independently from the floor; willingness and ability of parent or legal guardian to give informed consent; willingness and ability to comply with scheduled visits, drug administration plan, and study procedures; and ability to maintain reproducible FVC measurements.

The study is funded by the National Institutes of Health (Kate Bushby and Robert Griggs, study Chairs), and will begin enrollment in 2012.

DEVELOPMENT OF DISSOCIATIVE STEROIDS FOR DMD

An alternative approach to optimizing dosing regimens of traditional glucocorticoid drugs is to change the chemistry of the drug, with the goal of broadening the therapeutic window (increasing efficacy while decreasing side effects). Glucocorticoid drugs are recognized to have 2 subactivities: serving as a ligand for steroid hormone receptors, and nonreceptor-mediated effects on plasma membranes. The ligand/receptor complex has 2 further subactivities: transactivation and transrepression properties. Transactivation (also termed *cis*-regulation) is the best characterized molecular response, whereby ligand/glucocorticoid receptor complexes translocate from the cytoplasm to the nucleus and then interact directly with DNA and gene promoters (**Fig. 2**). With transactivation, the ligand/receptor dimers typically bind to a DNA sequence motif (glucocorticoid response elements [GRE]), and activate transcription of the nearby gene (hence the designation "transactivation"). Of importance, there is increasing evidence that the transactivation subactivity is associated more with side effects rather than with drug efficacy.[27]

Clinical efficacy, on the other hand, is increasingly associated with the second, transrepression subactivity. Transrepression involves ligand/receptor interactions with other cellular signaling proteins, such as nuclear factor (NF)-κB, activator protein 1, and STAT5 complexes, with downstream changes in cell signaling, and more indirect effects on gene transcription (non–GRE-mediated).[27,28] Transrepression has been associated with anti-inflammatory activity and clinical efficacy.

All steroid hormones, including glucocorticoids, are lipophilic, and readily traverse lipid bilayers (cell membranes). Some steroid drugs have been optimized for membrane activities, such as the lazaroids (see **Fig. 1**). Lazaroids, including the Δ-9,11 modification thought to block binding of the drug to the receptor, were optimized for effects on cell membranes (prevention of lipid peroxidation), and tested clinically for neuroprotection.[29–31] In DMD, there are well-documented changes in myofiber

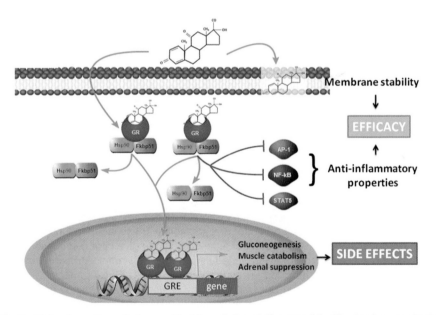

Fig. 2. Molecular action of glucocorticoids and dissociative steroids. Classic pharmacologic glucocorticoids have anti-inflammatory, membrane fluidity, and glucocorticoid response element (GRE)-mediated transcriptional activities. Dissociative steroids retain membrane and anti-inflammatory subactivities associated with efficacy, but do not retain the GRE-mediated transcriptional activities associated with side-effect profiles. GR, glucocorticoid receptor.

membrane function and integrity, and steroids are likely to modify this defect (for better or worse). Consistent with this, recent studies of lazaroids in myogenic cells in culture[32] and ischemia/reperfusion injury in vivo have shown benefit of lazaroid drugs.[33]

In an effort to improve upon glucocorticoid therapy for DMD, the authors studied drugs with the Δ-9,11 chemistry (see **Fig. 1**). The goal was to determine whether this chemistry represented a dissociative steroid (eg, separation of the transactivation [side effects] and transrepression [efficacy]) (see **Fig. 2**). A Δ-9,11 drug, anecortave, did in fact bind the glucocorticoid receptor, albeit at lower affinity than pharmacologic glucocorticoids.[34] Of importance, the ligand/glucocorticoid receptor complex was found to translocate to the nucleus, but showed no activity in binding to GRE elements and activating GRE-mediated gene transcription. Thus, the Δ-9,11 drug appeared to have lost the transactivation subactivity associated with many deleterious side effects (see **Fig. 2**).

To determine whether the Δ-9,11 drug retained transrepression (the subactivity associated with glucocorticoid efficacy), the authors studied anti-inflammatory effects using NF-κB reporter assays.[35] NF-κB inhibitory activity was found to be retained by the Δ-9,11 drug, at a potency similar to that of prednisone.[34] We were also interested in the effects of the drugs on the phospholipids that make up the membrane. Phospholipid bilayers have a hydrophilic head on the inner and outer walls of the membrane and hydrophobic tails. Lipids such as cholesterol are known to compress head groups, strengthen the bilayer, and decrease permeability when incorporated into a lipid bilayer. Indeed, our delta 9,11 steroids exert a similar and more profound effect on phospholipid bilayers than either prednisolone or cholesterol. The D-ring functionality (17-hydroxy-20-keto-21-hydroxy) orients within the phospholipid head groups while the hydrophobic ABC and most of the D ring orients in the lipid core. Since the C-17 C-20 bond can rotate, our compounds are operationally cone-like wedges in the phospholipid. They compress the head groups and decrease permeability while disordering the hydrophobic core which, among other things, protects against lipid peroxidation by decreasing the repeat number in lipid peroxidation chain reactions. This phenomenon for the delta 9,11 steroids has been described.[36] These results encouraged the authors to conduct a preclinical study of the dystrophin-deficient *mdx* mouse model of DMD. Evidence of efficacy in vivo was found, whereby daily oral delivery of Δ-9,11 analogue reduced muscle inflammation and improved multiple functional assays. Of note, no side effects of reductions in body weight or spleen size seen with prednisone treatment were observed, suggesting that the Δ-9,11 drug had indeed lost side effects. These data suggest that the Δ-9,11 chemistry holds promise as a dissociative steroid, with retention of efficacy via transrepression, and loss of side effects via reductions in transactivation subactivities. Current studies are focused on testing a series of Δ-9,11 compounds to optimize the potency, bioavailability, and toxicity profiles (lead compound selection), as well as testing of the optimized lead compound in animal models of multiple chronic inflammatory conditions, including other types of muscular dystrophy.

SUMMARY

DMD is among the most common of the muscular dystrophies, leading to shortened life span and considerable disability. Glucocorticoids are considered the standard of care, yet dose regimens have not been optimized, and the balance of efficacy and side effects for specific types of glucocorticoids requires further study. The FOR-DMD trial promises to shed light on dose optimization, as well as the therapeutic window of prednisone versus deflazacort. An alternative approach to optimizing currently available steroid regimens is to develop new drugs that are able to broaden the therapeutic window (increased efficacy with decreased side effects). Initial studies of Δ-9,11 modifications of the steroid backbone suggests that this chemistry produces a dissociative steroid, whereby anti-inflammatory activity is retained (transrepression) and membrane stabilization properties enhanced, while side effects are mitigated (loss of transactivation subactivity). Current studies are focusing on lead compound optimization using transactivation and membrane stability assays.

ACKNOWLEDGMENTS

The project described is supported by grant number U01NS061799 from the National Institute of Neurological Disorders and Stroke and U54HD053177 from the National Institute for Child Health and Human Development. The content is solely the responsibility of the authors and does not necessarily represent the official views of the National Institute of Neurological Disorders and Stroke, National Institute of Child Health and Human Development, or the National Institutes of Health. The authors acknowledge funding to TREAT-NMD by the EU FP6. Newcastle upon Tyne is a partner in the MRC Centre for Neuromuscular Diseases. ReveraGen receives funding from the National Institutes of Health TRND program of the National Center for Advancing Clinical Sciences, the Muscular Dystrophy Association Venture Philanthropy Fund, the US Department of Defense CDRMP, and Foundation to Eradicate Duchenne (FED).

REFERENCES

1. Hoffman EP, Brown RH, Kunkel LM. Dystrophin: the protein product of the Duchenne muscular dystrophy locus. Cell 1987;51:919–28.
2. Koenig M, Hoffman EP, Bertelson CJ, et al. Complete cloning of the Duchenne muscular dystrophy (DMD) cDNA and preliminary genomic organization of the DMD gene in normal and affected individuals. Cell 1987;50:509–17.
3. Angelini C, Pegoraro E, Turella E, et al. Deflazacort in Duchenne dystrophy: study of long-term effect. Muscle Nerve 1994;17(4):386–91.
4. Biggar WD, Harris VA, Eliasoph L, et al. Long-term benefits of deflazacort treatment for boys with Duchenne muscular dystrophy in their second decade. Neuromuscul Disord 2006;16:249–55.
5. Griggs RC, Moxley RT III, Mendell JR, et al. Prednisone in Duchenne dystrophy: a randomized, controlled trial defining the time course and dose response: Clinical Investigation of Duchenne Dystrophy Group. Arch Neurol 1991;48:383–8.
6. Griggs RC, Moxley RT III, Mendell JR, et al. Duchenne dystrophy: randomized, controlled trial of prednisone (18 months) and azathioprine (12 months). Neurology 1993;43:520–7.
7. Manzur AY, Kuntzer T, Pike M, et al. Glucocorticoid corticosteroids for Duchenne muscular dystrophy. Cochrane Database Syst Rev 2008;(1):CD003725.
8. Markham LW, Kinnett K, Wong BL, et al. Corticosteroid treatment retards development of ventricular dysfunction in Duchenne muscular dystrophy. Neuromuscul Disord 2008;18:365–70.
9. Mendell JR, Moxley RT, Griggs RC, et al. Randomized, double-blind six-month trial of prednisone in Duchenne's muscular dystrophy. N Engl J Med 1989;320:1592–7.
10. Moxley RT III, Ashwal S, Pandya S, et al. Practice parameter: corticosteroid treatment of Duchenne dystrophy: report of the Quality Standards Subcommittee of

the American Academy of Neurology and the Practice Committee of the Child Neurology Society. Neurology 2005;64:13–20.

11. Bushby K, Finkel R, Birnkrant DJ, et al. Diagnosis and management of Duchenne muscular dystrophy, part 1: diagnosis, and pharmacological and psychosocial management. Lancet Neurol 2010;9:77–93.

12. Bushby K, Finkel R, Birnkrant DJ, et al. Diagnosis and management of Duchenne muscular dystrophy, part 2: implementation of multidisciplinary care. Lancet Neurol 2010;9:177–89.

13. Connolly AM, Schierbecker J, Renna R, et al. High dose weekly oral prednisone improves strength in boys with Duchenne muscular dystrophy. Neuromuscul Disord 2002;12:917–25.

14. Escolar DM, Hache LP, Clemens PR, et al. Randomized, blinded trial of weekend vs daily prednisone in Duchenne muscular dystrophy. Neurology 2011;77(5): 444–52.

15. Brooke MH, Fenichel GM, Griggs RC, et al. Clinical investigation of Duchenne muscular dystrophy: interesting results in a trial of prednisone. Arch Neurol 1987;44:812–7.

16. Fenichel GM, Mendell JR, Moxley RT III, et al. A comparison of daily and alternate-day prednisone therapy in the treatment of Duchenne muscular dystrophy. Arch Neurol 1991;48:575–9.

17. Beenakker EA, Fock JM, Van Tol MJ, et al. Intermittent prednisone therapy in Duchenne muscular dystrophy: a randomized controlled trial. Arch Neurol 2005;62:128–32.

18. Sansome A, Royston P, Dubowitz V. Steroids in Duchenne muscular dystrophy: pilot study of a new low-dosage schedule. Neuromuscul Disord 1993;3:567–9.

19. Matthews DJ, James KA, Miller LA, et al, MD STARnet. Use of corticosteroids in a population-based cohort of boys with Duchenne and Becker muscular dystrophy. J Child Neurol 2010;25(11):1319–24.

20. Angelini C. The role of corticosteroids in muscular dystrophy: a critical appraisal. Muscle Nerve 2007;36(4):424–35.

21. Schara U, Mortier J, Mortier W. Long-term steroid therapy in Duchenne muscular dystrophy-positive results versus side effects. J Clin Neuromuscul Dis 2001;2(4): 179–83.

22. Pereira RM, Freire de Carvalho J. Glucocorticoid-induced myopathy. Joint Bone Spine 2011;78(1):41–4.

23. Hoffman EP, Nader GA. Balancing muscle hypertrophy and atrophy. Nat Med 2004 Jun;10(6):584–5.

24. Mesa LE, Dubrovsky AL, Corderi J, et al. Steroids in Duchenne muscular dystrophy—deflazacort trial. Neuromuscul Disord 1991;1(4):261–6.

25. Bonifati MD, Ruzza G, Bonometto P, et al. A multicenter, double-blind, randomized trial of deflazacort versus prednisone in Duchenne muscular dystrophy. Muscle Nerve 2000;23(9):1344–7.

26. Biggar WD, Politano L, Harris VA, et al. Deflazacort in Duchenne muscular dystrophy: a comparison of two different protocols. Neuromuscul Disord 2004; 14(8–9):476–82.

27. Newton R, Holden NS. Separating transrepression and transactivation: a distressing divorce for the glucocorticoid receptor? Mol Pharmacol 2007;72:799–809.

28. Rhen T, Cidlowski JA. Anti-inflammatory action of glucocorticoids—new mechanisms for old drugs. N Engl J Med 2005;353:1711–23.

29. Taylor BM, Fleming WE, Benjamin CW, et al. The mechanism of cytoprotective action of lazaroids I: Inhibition of reactive oxygen species formation and lethal

cell injury during periods of energy depletion. J Pharmacol Exp Ther 1996;276: 1224–31.

30. Bracken MB, Shephard MJ, Holford TR, et al. Administration of methylprednisolone for 24 or 48 h or tirilazadmesylate for 48 h in the treatment of acute spinal cord injury; results of the third national acute spinal cord injury randomized controlled trial. JAMA 1997;277:1597–604.

31. Kavanagh RJ, Kam PC. Lazaroids: efficacy and mechanism of action of the 21-aminosteroids in neuroprotection. Br J Anaesth 2001;86:110–9.

32. Passaquin AC, Lhote P, Rüegg UT. Calcium influx inhibition by steroids and analogs in C2C12 skeletal muscle cells. Br J Pharmacol 1998;124:1751–9.

33. Campo GM, Squadrito F, Campo S, et al. Antioxidant activity of U-83836E, a second generation lazaroid, during myocardial ischemia/reperfusion injury. Free Radic Res 1997;27:577–90.

34. Baudy AR, Reeves E, Damsker JM, et al. Δ-9, 11 modification of glucocorticoids dissociate NF-κB inhibitory efficacy from GRE-associated side effects. J Pharmacol Exp Ther 2012;343:225–32.

35. Baudy AR, Saxena N, Gordish H, et al. A robust in vitro screening assay to identify NF-kappaB inhibitors for inflammatory muscle diseases. Int Immunopharmacol 2009;9:1209–14.

36. Epps DE, McCall JM. Physical and Chemical Mechanisms of the Antioxidant Action of Tirilazad Mesylate in Handbook of Novel Antioxidants. Antioxid Health Dis 1997;4:95–137.

Management of Pulmonary Complications in Neuromuscular Disease

Lisa F. Wolfe, MD[a], Nanette C. Joyce, DO[b],*, Craig M. McDonald, MD[b], Joshua O. Benditt, MD[c], Jonathan Finder, MD[d]

KEYWORDS

- Restrictive lung disease • Nocturnal hypoventilation • Noninvasive ventilation
- Pulmonary function test • Respiratory failure

KEY POINTS

- Restrictive lung disease occurs commonly in patients with neuromuscular disease.
- The earliest sign of respiratory compromise in the patient with neuromuscular disease is nocturnal hypoventilation, which progresses over time to include daytime hypoventilation and eventually the need for full-time mechanical ventilation.
- Pulmonary function testing should be done during regular follow-up visits to identify the need for assistive respiratory equipment and initiate early noninvasive ventilation.
- Initiation of noninvasive ventilation can improve quality of life and prolong survival in patients with neuromuscular disease.

INTRODUCTION

Normal breathing depends on the intact function of the ventilator pump, which consists of the central respiratory control centers, the bony rib cage, and the muscles of breathing. In progressive neuromuscular diseases (NMDs), the ventilator pump is often impaired and leads to a predictable pattern of respiratory compromise beginning with normal or near normal unassisted gas exchange early in the disease, adequate daytime gas exchange with nocturnal hypoventilation during mid-stage disease, and chronic and/or acute respiratory failure requiring full-time assisted ventilatory support for survival in late-stage disease. In addition, normal defense of the lung depends on adequate secretion management and the precise timing of and force generated by the

[a] Division of Pulmonary and Critical Care Medicine, Northwestern University Feinberg School of Medicine, McGaw Pavilion, Suite M-300, 240 East Huron Street, Chicago, IL 60611, USA; [b] Department of Physical Medicine and Rehabilitation, School of Medicine, University of California Davis, 4860 Y Street, Suite 3850, Sacramento, CA 95822, USA; [c] University of Washington Medical Center, 1959 North East Pacific Street, Seattle, WA 98195, USA; [d] Children's Hospital of Pittsburgh of UPMC, Administration Office Building, Suite 3300, 4401 Penn Avenue, Suite Floor 3, Pittsburgh, PA 15224, USA
* Corresponding author.
E-mail address: Nanette.joyce@ucdmc.ucdavis.edu

Phys Med Rehabil Clin N Am 23 (2012) 829–853
http://dx.doi.org/10.1016/j.pmr.2012.08.010
1047-9651/12/$ – see front matter © 2012 Published by Elsevier Inc.

activities of the ventilator pump to produce an effective cough. Pneumonia, respiratory failure, and, ultimately, death can all occur as a consequence of ventilator pump dysfunction. For many NMDs, breathing disorders are recognized as the leading cause of mortality.[1,2] However, appropriate screening with timely intervention and use of assistive respiratory devices can prevent complications and prolong life in those in whom NMD compromises their respiratory system.[2–4]

CAUSE OF RESPIRATORY FAILURE IN NMD
Normal Breathing

Breathing is an active, primarily involuntary process requiring work. Inspiration occurs as the diaphragm and external intercostal muscles contract and expand the thorax, causing the intrapulmonary pressure to decrease and pull air into the lungs. Air enters the upper airway against resistance and travels via bulk flow, like a water faucet, through to the terminal bronchioles. As the cross-sectional area of the lung dramatically increases in the respiratory zone, the alveolated region of the lung, the forward velocity of air dramatically slows and diffusion becomes the chief mode of ventilation. After air exchange, quiet exhalation occurs passively, propelled by energy stored during inspiration from the elastic properties of the tissues of the rib cage and lung. The recoil of the rib cage and lung tissues increases intrapulmonary pressure, reverses airflow, and expels CO_2 abundant air from the lungs. During stressed breathing, the elastic recoil is not sufficient to cause rapid expiration and the abdominal and internal intercostals participate.

The work of breathing depends on both the elastic and viscous forces of the lung. Under normal conditions, the work of breathing is quite small and requires less than 5% of total resting O_2 consumption. In restrictive lung physiology caused by NMD, however, the work of breathing increases. Respiratory failure results from several factors that either increase or are influenced by the increased work of breathing, including (1) respiratory muscle weakness and fatigue, (2) alteration in respiratory system mechanics, and (3) impairment of the central control of respiration.

Respiratory Muscle Weakness and Fatigue

Respiratory muscle weakness and fatigue are frequent contributors to ventilator failure in the patient with NMD. Respiratory muscle *weakness,* the inability of the respiratory muscles to generate normal levels of pressure and flow during inspiration or expiration, occurs because of lack of appropriate neural stimulation of muscle fibers, as in spinal cord injury and amyotrophic lateral sclerosis (ALS), or intrinsic muscle disease, as in the muscular dystrophies. Weakness of the muscles of inspiration (the diaphragm, intercostals, and accessory muscles) results in inadequate lung expansion, with subsequent microatelectasis, leading to ventilation/perfusion mismatch and consequent hypoxemia. Compensatory tachypnea, with small tidal volumes, exacerbates the atelectasis and further reduces the compliance of the respiratory system, increasing the mechanical load on already weakened respiratory muscles.[4] Progressive muscle weakness and fatigue lead to restrictive lung disease with hypoventilation, hypercarbia, and respiratory failure. As opposed to the chronic progressive changes in pulmonary function caused by respiratory muscle weakness, respiratory muscle fatigue causing ventilator failure usually occurs after impairment of respiratory muscle strength has been reduced to 30% of predicted values.[5]

Measures of respiratory muscle strength

There is continued investigation into the best measures of respiratory muscle strength for the patient with NMD and how these measures offer prognostic information and predict onset of nocturnal hypoxemia and respiratory failure. Historically, the maximal inspiratory pressure (MIP) and maximal expiratory pressure (MEP) have been used as measures of respiratory strength. Several studies have identified the sniff nasal inspiratory pressure (SNIP) as a consistent measure with good prognostic value in patients with NMDs. In ALS, the SNIP showed greater consistency across disease severity compared with forced vital capacity (FVC), MIP, or MEP in patients with severe bulbar dysfunction.[6,7] Studies have demonstrated a linear decline in SNIP as ALS progresses and a strong correlation between low SNIP measure and nocturnal hypoxemia.[6,7] In a study of 98 patients with ALS, an SNIP of less than 40 cm H_2O had a sensitivity of 97% and a specificity of 79% for death within 6 months.[7]

Spirometry with FVC measurement has been commonly used as a measure of respiratory strength and function. Supine positioning eliminates the affects of gravity and may be a better marker of diaphragmatic strength, and in ALS, supine FVC is the best predictor of survival.[8,9] Spirometry alone is not sufficient to predict early physiologic respiratory failure with nocturnal hypoventilation. In the setting of Duchenne muscular dystrophy (DMD), FVC values have no ability to predict nocturnal elevation in end-tidal CO_2.[10]

What has become clear is that there is no single screening test that can accurately predict the development of nocturnal hypoventilation or survival. Multiple modalities testing has been shown to be a more effective strategy.[11,12] In DMD, a forced expiratory volume in 1 second of less than 40% predicted, a $Paco_2$ 45 mm Hg or greater, and a base excess greater than 4 mmol/L are factors that indicate the development of sleep-disordered breathing.[11] In ALS, the use of 5 tests at each visit allowed for early initiation of noninvasive ventilation (NIV) and was associated with improved survival. The panel of tests included upright and supine FVC, upright and supine MIP, and overnight oximetry.[12]

When using lung function testing to assess cough and need for airway clearance, the mentioned testing strategy has not been as effective. Peak cough flow testing using a peak flowmeter instead of a spirometer can accurately predict the need to initiate airway clearance (<270 L/min) or the potential need for tracheotomy (<160 L/min).[13]

Alteration in Respiratory Mechanics

In addition to effects on muscle contraction, NMD increases elastic and resistive loads on the respiratory muscles. Both types of loads increase the work of breathing and hasten ventilator failure. Increases in elastic loads are a consequence of abnormal stiffness of both the lungs[14] and the chest wall.[15,16] Finally, kyphoscoliosis, which is frequently associated with NMD, results in deformation of the thoracic cage, altering the biomechanics of the respiratory muscles and compromising their ability to operate effectively against the increased elastic and resistive loads, further increasing the work of breathing.[14] Thoracolumbar scoliosis is almost universal in boys, with DMD with the most profound effect on ventilation occurring in those in whom the curves have an early onset. Vital capacity may be disproportionately reduced in this case, but even in adolescents with severe scoliosis, the impact on vital capacity is correlated with the magnitude of the curve.[17-20]

Impairment of Control of Ventilation

Disorders of central control of respiration frequently are associated with NMD processes. Defects in control of respiration may be caused by central factors as in bulbar poliomyelitis or ALS. Central factors associated with control of ventilation during sleep impact respiratory function even in primarily muscular disorders. The first indicator of disordered respiratory control typically occurs in association with sleep. The supine sleep position increases work of breathing by increasing resistance from the chest and abdomen. Slow-wave sleep reduces both tidal volume and respiratory rate, whereas stage rapid eye movement further stresses the system by causing atonia in accessory muscles. In a system already stressed, these changes can drive the development of hypoventilation with hypoxemia and CO_2 retention.[21]

Symptoms and signs of nocturnal hypoventilation include air hunger, snoring, choking, orthopnea, cyanosis, restlessness, insomnia, daytime hypersomnolence, morning headaches, drowsiness, fatigue, depression, and impaired cognition.[22] Significant nocturnal decreases in partial pressure of oxygen (Pao_2) and elevations in arterial partial pressure of carbon dioxide ($Paco_2$) have been reported.[23–26] These changes most commonly begin to occur during rapid eye movement sleep when a pattern of rapid shallow breathing develops as a result of supraspinal inhibition of the alpha motor neuron drive, maximizing hypotonia to prevent motor activity during dreams.[23–26] Nocturnal hypoventilation sometimes is associated with apneic episodes, leading to additional hypercapnia.[24,25,27] Hypercapnia or hypoxemia occurring at night may have a role in reducing daytime central respiratory drive by depressing central drive centers directly and by increasing the "bicarbonate pool."[24,25,28] This latter effect blunts the stimulus to increase respiratory rate generated by respiratory acidosis and perpetuates the hypercapnic state. In addition, as the work of breathing increases, patients with restrictive lung disease reach a threshold at which increasing $Paco_2$ will no longer drive the homeostatic response to increase respiratory rate and CO_2 accumulates.[21]

Presentation of Respiratory Failure and Variable Practice Patterns Regarding Management

Respiratory failure typically present in 1 of 3 ways in patients with NMD: (1) as acute respiratory failure such as that occurring in high-level spinal cord injury, Guillain-Barre syndrome, and tick paralysis; (2) as an acute respiratory decompensation in a chronic disease such as ALS or myasthenia gravis; or (3) as a chronic worsening of a gradually progressive disease such as DMD.

Treatment of acute respiratory failure frequently involves endotracheal intubation and positive pressure ventilation (PPV) in the intensive care unit. Often tracheostomy tube placement is required. In this situation, unfortunately, there are few choices of methods of ventilation. Under certain circumstances, it is possible to wean a patient from invasive PPV by using a variety of noninvasive ventilator techniques.[29] Thus, the tracheostomy tube, which some patients find objectionable, is not necessarily permanent.

The more common presentation, with insidious onset of respiratory failure in patients with NMD, can be improved by early intervention to prevent respiratory complications and prolong life. Noninvasive forms of both positive and negative ventilation and the rocking bed have been used effectively in reversing, at least temporarily, progressive chronic respiratory failure.[30–33] Initially, patients may require ventilator support for only part of the day. In these cases, nocturnal ventilatory support has been shown to be of great value.[30,32–36] Daytime ventilation either full-time or for prescribed periods can be used as muscular weakness progresses. Thus, monitoring a patient's pulmonary function becomes of paramount importance in directing treatment. A survey of ALS clinic directors published in 1999 was a focused query to determine common pulmonary practices.[37] This study found that 85% of ALS clinics performed pulmonary function tests (PFTs) every 3 months during clinic visits and decisions to initiate NIV were based on PFT results. Despite this, a later study revealed that only 15.9% of patients with ALS were using therapy with NIV.[38]

Development of Consensus Guidelines for Pulmonary Management of NMDs

Several consensus practice parameters have been developed to outline disease-specific pulmonary monitoring and management recommendations.

ALS

A consensus statement, based on a systematic review of the literature, was recently published with recommendations for pulmonary management in ALS.[2] The American Academy of Neurology (AAN) consensus document acknowledges that management of the patient with ALS is best accomplished with multispecialty care teams. Respiratory care providers play a key role in these teams. Their focus includes 3 areas: (1) lung function assessment, (2) prevention of chest infections, and (3) ventilatory support.

Lung function assessment is used to help in the timing of percutaneous endoscopic gastrostomy tube (PEG) placement, initiation of NIV, and considerations for end-of-life care. Nutritional support has been found to be beneficial in improving survival and quality of life for both patients and care-givers. The placement of PEG tubes includes risk resulting from anesthetic and procedural complications such as aspiration, pneumonia, and ventilator failure. The lower the lung function, the greater is the risk of the procedure. The AAN recommendations suggest PEG placement at an FVC greater than 50% and placement should be performed with great caution if the FVC is less than 30%.

When using lung function testing to assess need to initiate NIV, the AAN guidelines discuss the use of testing with an MIP greater than –60, SNP less than 40, or FVC less than 50% as the time to initiate therapy (**Fig. 1**). The guidelines from Centers for Medicare and Medicaid Services have additional suggestions for initiation of NIV including oxygen saturation of 88% or less for longer than 5 minutes or a $Paco_2$ less than 45.[38] Last, the AAN guidelines suggest the use of lung function testing to assess survival. Survival of less than 3 months is noted with SNIP of less than 30 cm H_2O. Daytime saturation less than 95% or nocturnal saturation less than 93% had similar findings.

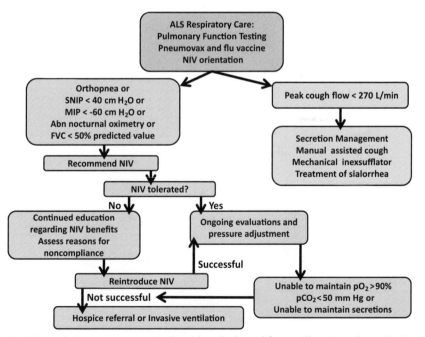

Fig. 1. ALS respiratory management algorithm. (*Adapted from* Miller RG, Jackson CE, Kasarskis EJ, et al. Practice parameter update: the care of the patient with amyotrophic lateral sclerosis: drug, nutritional, and respiratory therapies (an evidence-based review): report of the Quality Standards Subcommittee of the American Academy of Neurology. Neurology 2009;73:1218–26; with permission.)

The AAN recommends a proactive approach to prevent chest infections as these represent a high source of morbidity and mortality in the ALS patient group. The AAN recommends performing vaccination with both pneumovax and influenza vaccination. Airway clearance techniques should be initiated when the peak cough flow testing is less than 270 L/min. Artificial cough support is most strongly recommended using a mechanical inexsufflation (MIE) device (**Fig. 2**). These devices support both the inhale and exhale components of cough with delivery of positive pressure followed by negative pressure through either a mask or mouthpiece. Although there are limited data, the use of high-frequency chest wall oscillation may be beneficial. These devices, wrapped around the torso, provide vibratory force through the chest wall to the lung to help keep mucus mobile, preventing atelectasis (**Fig. 3**). Nebulized medications are frequently used in conjunction with these techniques but there are no data to support their use.

Ventilation is strongly supported. NIV is recommended to both improve disease outcomes and improve the quality of life for both patients and care-givers. There are no specific recommendations as to the type of NIV device or settings to be used. It should be noted, however, that the recommendations from the Centers for Medicare and Medicaid Services suggest the use of an NIV device with a back-up rate instead of a spontaneous breathing device.[39] Tracheostomy with mechanical ventilation (TIV) is suggested in the AAN guidelines, as it has been shown to have equal quality of life and acceptance by patients compaired to NIV. Those with cognitive impairment, bulbar disease, or lowest lung function are more likely to require TIV.

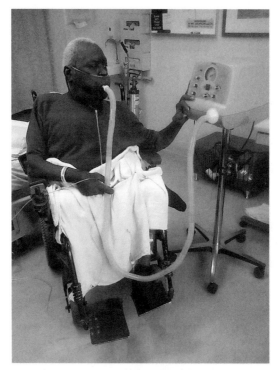

Fig. 2. Patient using a mechanical inexsufflator (MIE) for airway clearance. The interface pictured is a mouthpiece;options include a facemask and an adapter for use with a tracheotomy.

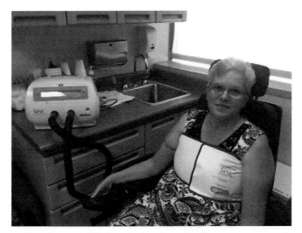

Fig. 3. High frequency chest oscillation device for secretion management.

DMD

In 2004, the American Thoracic Society published guidelines for respiratory care in DMD. Their recommendations were as follows: Each child with confirmed DMD should undergo an evaluation of respiratory status early (between ages 4 and 6), and tests of respiratory function should be performed at every clinic visit thereafter. Regular cardiac evaluations should start at school age and patients should be seen by a pulmonologist twice a year beginning at age 12 or when their FVC deteriorates to 80% of normal. Care by a pulmonologist should be increased to every 3 to 6 months after the initiation of assisted ventilation or an airway clearance device. Cough effectiveness should be evaluated regularly, and patients should be instructed on the use of a manual cough assist maneuver or an assisted coughing device, as well as taught how to use an oximeter at home to measure blood oxygen levels. Last, these recommendations addressed the importance of maintaining good nutrition with use of a gastrostomy tube if necessary.[40]

In 2010, the Centers for Disease Control and Prevention (CDC) sponsored the development of consensus care considerations for DMD using experts in multiple disciplines including pediatric and adult pulmonary medicine. A RAND methodology was used.

The aim of respiratory care is to allow timely prevention and management of complications. The experts concluded that a structured, proactive approach to respiratory management that includes use of assisted cough and nocturnal ventilation has been shown to prolong survival.[41–43] Patients with DMD are at risk of respiratory complications as their condition deteriorates as a result of progressive loss of respiratory muscle strength, including ineffective cough,[13,44–50] nocturnal hypoventilation, sleep disordered breathing, and, ultimately, daytime respiratory failure.[11,24,51–57]

The care team must include a physician and therapist with skill in the initiation and management of NIV and associated interfaces,[58–64] lung-volume recruitment techniques,[65–67] and manual and mechanically assisted cough.[68–75]

Assessments and interventions will need to be reevaluated as the patient's condition changes (**Tables 1–3**).[3] In the ambulatory stage, minimum assessment of pulmonary function (eg, measurement of FVC at least annually) allows familiarity with the equipment and the team can assess the maximum respiratory function achieved. The main need for pulmonary care is in the period after the loss of independent ambulation. A respiratory action plan should be enacted with increasing disease severity.[76]

Although the expert panel recognized that assisted ventilation via tracheostomy can prolong survival, the care considerations advocate strongly for the use of noninvasive

Table 1
CDC DMD care considerations workgroup recommendations regarding respiratory assessment (in the clinic) of patients with DMD

DMD Patient Status	Recommended Clinical Assessments	Assessment Frequency
Ages $\geq$6 y: Ambulatory	Sitting FVC	No less than annual evaluation
Non-ambulatory	Spo$_2$ PFTs: • Sitting FVC • Peak cough flow Optional measures: • MIP • MEP	No less than every 6 mo
Nonambulatory with: • Suspected hypoventilation • FVC <50% predicted • Use of assisted ventilation	Capnography measuring: awake $_{ET}CO_2$	No less than annual evaluations and with each respiratory infection in a patient with FVC <50% predicted

Data from Bushby K, Finkel R, Birnkrant DJ, et al. Diagnosis and management of Duchenne muscular dystrophy, part 2: implementation of multidisciplinary care. Lancet Neurol 2010;9(2):177–89.

modes of assisted ventilation. Particular attention to respiratory status is required around the time of planned surgery.

Immunization with 23-valent pneumococcal polysaccharide vaccine is indicated for patients aged 2 years and older. Annual immunization with trivalent inactivated

Table 2
CDC DMD care considerations workgroup recommendations regarding respiratory assessment (at home) of patients with DMD

DMD Patient Status	Strongly Recommended Assessment
• If baseline peak cough flow is <270 L/min[a] and patient has an acute respiratory infection	Pulse oximetry
• When baseline peak cough flow is <160 L/min	Pulse oximetry
• Signs and symptoms of hypoventilation[b]	Measure gas exchange during sleep[c]
DMD patient status	Assessment to be strongly considered
• Baseline FVC <40% • Awake baseline blood or end-tidal CO_2 >45 mm Hg • Awake baseline Spo$_2$ <95% • FVC <1.25 L in any teenage or older patient	Measure gas exchange during sleep[a]

Abbreviation: Spo$_2$, pulse oximetry.

[a] All specified threshold values of peak cough flow and MEP apply to older teenage and adult patients.

[b] Signs/symptoms of hypoventilation include fatigue, dyspnea, morning or continuous headaches, sleep dysfunction (frequent nocturnal awakenings [>3], difficult arousal), hypersomnolence, awakenings with dyspnea and tachycardia, difficulty with concentration, frequent nightmares.

[c] Dual-channel oximetry-capnography in the home is strongly recommended, but other recommended methods include home oximetry during sleep and polysomnography, the method of choice being determined by local availability, expertise, and clinician preference.

Data from Bushby K, Finkel R, Birnkrant DJ, et al. Diagnosis and management of Duchenne muscular dystrophy, part 2: implementation of multidisciplinary care. Lancet Neurol 2010;9(2):177–89.

Table 3
Respiratory interventions indicated in patients with DMD

Step 1: volume recruitment/deep lung inflation technique	Volume recruitment/deep lung inflation technique (by self-inflating manual ventilation bag or mechanical insufflation–exsufflation) when FVC <40% predicted
Step 2: manual and mechanically assisted cough techniques	Necessary when: • Respiratory infection present and baseline peak cough flow <270 L/min[a] • Baseline peak cough flow <160 L/min or MEP <40 cm H_2O • Baseline FVC <40% predicted or <1.25 L in older teenager/adult
Step 3: nocturnal ventilation	Nocturnal ventilation[b] is indicated in patients who have any of the following: • Signs or symptoms of hypoventilation (patients with FVC <30% predicted are at especially high risk) • A baseline Spo_2 <95% and/or blood or end-tidal CO_2 >45 mm Hg while awake • An apnea–hypopnea index >10/h on polysomnography or ≥4 episodes of Spo_2 <92% or drops in Spo_2 of ≥4% per hour of sleep Optimally, use of lung volume recruitment and assisted cough techniques should always precede initiation of NIV
Step 4: daytime ventilation	In patients already using nocturnally assisted ventilation, daytime ventilation[c] is indicated for: • Self-extension of nocturnal ventilation into waking hours • Abnormal deglutition caused by dyspnea, which is relieved by ventilatory assistance • Inability to speak a full sentence without breathlessness and/or • Symptoms of hypoventilation with baseline Spo_2 <95% and/or blood or end-tidal CO_2 >45 mm Hg while awake Continuous noninvasive assisted ventilation (with mechanically assisted cough) can facilitate endotracheal extubation for patients who were intubated during acute illness or during anesthesia, followed by weaning to nocturnal noninvasive assisted ventilation, if applicable
Step 5: tracheostomy	Indications for tracheostomy include: • Patient and clinician preference[d] • Patient cannot successfully use NIV • Inability of the local medical infrastructure to support NIV • Three failures to achieve extubation during critical illness despite optimum use of NIV and mechanically assisted cough • The failure of noninvasive methods of cough assistance to prevent aspiration of secretions into the lung and drops in oxygen saturation <95% or the patient's baseline, necessitating frequent direct tracheal suctioning via tracheostomy

Abbreviation: Spo_2, pulse oximetry.

[a] All specified threshold values of peak cough flow and MEP apply to older teenage and adult patients.

[b] Recommended for nocturnal use: NIV with pressure-cycled bilevel devices or volume-cycled ventilators or combination volume-pressure ventilators. In bilevel or pressure support modes of ventilation, add a back-up rate of breathing. Recommended interfaces include a nasal mask or a nasal pillow. Other interfaces can be used and each has its own potential benefits.

[c] Recommended for day use: NIV with portable volume-cycled or volume-pressure ventilators; bilevel devices are an alternative. A mouthpiece interface is strongly recommended during day use of portable volume-cycled or volume-pressure ventilators, but other ventilator-interface combinations can be used depending on clinician preference and patient comfort.

[d] However, the panel advocates the long-term use of NIV up to and including 24 h/d in eligible patients.

Data from Bushby K, Finkel R, Birnkrant DJ, et al. Diagnosis and management of Duchenne muscular dystrophy, part 2: implementation of multidisciplinary care. Lancet Neurol 2010;9(2):177–89.

influenza vaccine is indicated for patients 6 months of age and older. Neither the pneumococcal vaccine nor the influenza vaccine is a live vaccine, and thus they can be administered to patients treated with glucocorticoids, but the immune response to vaccination might be diminished. Up-to-date and detailed information on immunization indications, contraindications, and schedules can be obtained from various sources, including the American Academy of Pediatrics and the CDC.[3]

During an established infection, in addition to the use of manually and mechanically assisted cough, antibiotics are necessary, regardless of oxygen saturation if positive evidence of an infection is established on culture and regardless of culture results if pulse oximetry remains at less than 95% in room air.[3] Supplemental oxygen therapy should be used with caution because oxygen therapy can apparently improve hypoxemia while masking the underlying cause, such as atelectasis or hypoventilation. Oxygen therapy might impair central respiratory drive and exacerbate hypercapnia.[64,68,77] If a patient has hypoxemia as a result of hypoventilation, retained respiratory secretions, and/or atelectasis, then manual and mechanically assisted cough and NIV support are necessary. Substitution of these methods by oxygen therapy is dangerous.[43]

Spinal muscular atrophy

Similar to patients with other neuromuscuolar disorders, children with spinal muscular atrophy (SMA) are at high risk of pulmonary related morbidity and mortality. Notably, children with SMA have not only diaphragm weakness but also a more prominent issue with a greater involvement of expiratory and intercostal muscles. In SMA type 1 and type 2, this causes a bell-shaped chest and sternal deformity. In SMA type 3, kyphoscoliosis adds to the chest wall restriction issues.

Lung function assessment has not been well studied in SMA. Recommendations have been derived by expert opinion only.[77,78] There is a trend to adjust the type and frequency of lung function assessments by age and phenotype. Of those with SMA type 1, patients (nonsitters) are young and therefore unable to participate in standard lung function testing. High respiratory rates and paradoxic breathing are important physical examination findings. Pulse oximetry less than 94% supports a high likelihood of hypoventilation. Although many other tools are available and can be used, there are no formal recommendations for the frequency of use of transcutaneous CO_2, overnight oximetry, full polysomnography, chest radiography, or swallow evaluation. SMA type 2 patients (sitters) are similar to SMA type 1 patients except lung function testing becomes possible as the child ages and symptom assessment is easier. Symptoms should be used to drive assessment choices. SMA type 3 (walkers) patients have relatively late onset of respiratory failure – even into adulthood, but regular assessment with spirometry and polysomnography is recommended. The intervals for testing are not fixed and should be driven by symptom assessment.

Respiratory interventions should be driven by the integration of a pulmonary physician in to the formal SMA team. This professional will need to coordinate care for hospitalization, for instance, around a surgery or pneumonia. In addition, pulmonary support should ensure that preventative care is performed. such as immunizations.

Airway clearance on a routine basis is important as age appropriate and could include the use of the high-frequency chest wall oscillation, MIE, or nebulized medication. The family should be guided in an anticipatory manner to set very clear clinical goals with the pulmonary team member, addressing options for noninvasive, or invasive mechanical ventilation as well as alternatives for hospice care.

Congenital muscular dystrophies

Congenital myopathies are a large group of disorders that include many different genetic abnormalities and phenotypes. These disorders vary from other NMDs because muscle weakness alone is not responsible for respiratory impairment. Central nervous system lesions and cognitive dysfunction contribute to abnormalities in control of ventilation, swallowing, and cough. The presence of mutations including abnormalities in laminin, collagen, etc, can be present, causing scoliosis and/or spinal rigidity. The involvement of these structural elements can allow for respiratory failure to occur as a result of loss of spine and core rigidity, before the development of global weakness. As a group, these patients develop early-onset respiratory failure and require aggressive airway clearance and ventilator support. There are no trials that address these techniques directly in the setting of congenital myopathies. Expert consensus has recommended[79]:

- Perform full spirometry with every visit.
- Obtain one overnight oximetry examination if the patient shows an abnormal physical examination with increased work of breathing such as tachypnea or retractions. The patient may have signs of sleep disruption such as restlessness during sleep or decreased functioning during the day. Last, obtain overnight oximetry examination if there are recurrent chest infections, poor weight gain, morning headache, or FVC less than 60% or if a greater than 20% difference is observed between sitting and supine FVC if sitting FVC is less than 80%.
- Obtain one-night CO_2 monitoring if oximetry has a low baseline of less than 94% on room air when patient is awake or asleep and/or oximetry drops to less than 90% on room air for longer than 5 minutes with a low of at least 85% or greater than 30% of total sleep time spent at less than 90% saturation.
- Obtain a blood gas analysis if there is an acute onset of respiratory distress, if noninvasive CO_2 monitoring is not available, or to correlate with $ETCO_2$ and transcutaneous measurements obtained.
- Obtain one-night full polysomnogram (with end-tidal CO_2) for suspected gas exchange abnormalities caused by hypoventilation. Hypoventilation is present if greater than 25% of the total sleep time is spent with CO_2 greater than 50 mm Hg; also, polysomnography may be helpful to titrate best settings for NIV.

Respiratory considerations for patients with NMD undergoing general anesthesia and surgery

The CDC DMD Care Considerations Working group published specific respiratory management issues for patients undergoing general anesthesia and surgery. Respiratory interventions are intended to provide adequate respiratory support during induction of, maintenance of, and recovery from procedural sedation or general anesthesia. In particular, they are designed to reduce the risk of postprocedure endotracheal extubation failure, postoperative atelectasis, and pneumonia.[80] These goals can be achieved by providing noninvasively assisted ventilation and assisted cough after surgery for patients with significant respiratory-muscle weakness, as indicated by subthreshold preoperative PFT results.

Preoperative training in and postoperative use of NIV is strongly recommended for patients with a baseline FVC of less than 50% predicted and necessary with an FVC of less than 30% predicted.[81] Incentive spirometry is not indicated owing to potential lack of efficacy in patients with respiratory muscle weakness and the availability of preferred alternatives, such as mechanical insufflation–exsufflation. After careful consideration of the risks and benefits, patients with significant respiratory-muscle weakness might be eligible for surgery, albeit with increased risk, if these patients are highly skilled preoperatively in the use of NIV and assisted cough.[82,83]

METHODS OF VENTILATORY SUPPORT IN NMD
Mechanical Ventilation

Artificial ventilation as a means of prolonging human life has been referred to since Biblical times. As early as the mid-nineteenth century, ventilation during surgery, including open-chest operations, has been possible. It was not until 1927 and the invention of the motorized iron lung by Drinker that long-term mechanical ventilation became a possibility.[84] Chronic ventilation via a tracheostomy tube became possible in the 1950s with the development of reliable, smaller positive pressure ventilators. Today a wide variety of devices exist for chronic ventilation of patients with NMD and other forms of respiratory failure.

Negative pressure ventilators

Negative pressure ventilators have been used for many years, bringing extensive experience ventilating patients with a wide range of NMDs. Negative pressure ventilators function by applying a negative pressure to the surface of the thorax and abdomen, expanding the chest wall and lungs, and thus promoting the movement of air into the lungs. Exhalation occurs passively because of the inward elastic recoil of the chest wall and lungs. Because pleural pressure is lowered during inspiration, this type of ventilation more closely mimics spontaneous breathing than does PPV. Full body ventilators such as the iron lung encase the patient's entire body except for the head, which remains outside the device and is sealed at the neck with a rubber or plastic collar. Cyclic negative pressure is created within the tank by a bellows pump connected to an electric motor that can be powered by alternating current or a back-up battery supply. Respiratory rate and the volume of each breath can be adjusted. Because of the large size and weight (325 kg)[33] of the iron lung, the use of the iron lung is less practical and rarely used. Smaller and lighter devices have been developed and are still in use both in the United States and around the world.[85]

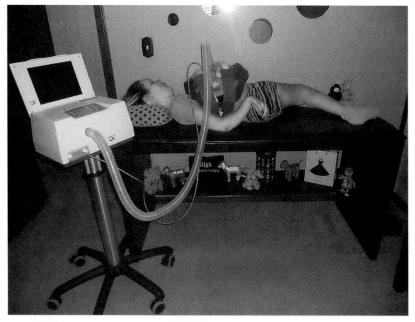

Fig. 4. Cuirass negative pressure ventilation device.

The cuirass or chest shell (**Fig. 4**) is a device that was developed to overcome the portability and confinement problems of the larger tank ventilators. It consists of a fiberglass shell that fits over the anterior chest and abdomen. This is attached to a negative pressure generator. Intermittent negative pressure is generated within the shell, resulting in expansion of the chest wall and lungs. Although portable and more convenient than the "full-body" negative pressure ventilators, the cuirass is the least efficient of the negative pressure ventilator devices.[86] The light weight and ease of application are attractive features of this device. Although the cuirass has been used for patients who require 24-hour ventilation, it probably is best reserved for those who require less ventilator assistance. The currently marketed device can also be used as an airway clearance device providing high-frequency oscillation and cough assist, as well as ventilatory support.[87]

Negative pressure ventilators, especially the more efficient types, have been used to continuously ventilate patients with little or no vital capacity.[35] The utility of negative pressure ventilators is limited because patients must be in the supine position when using them, and obese patients or those with significant kyphoscoliosis will require the use of a less portable option because the cuirass and wrap ventilators may not fit adequately. Travel is not possible with the larger devices. Finally, sleeping with a spouse or significant other is generally not possible with any of the devices.

One potential hazard of negative pressure mechanical ventilation is the development of upper airway obstruction during the negative pressure.[29,88] Airway collapse can occur with the negative intratracheal pressure generated by the ventilator is unopposed by upper airway muscle tone. This occurs most frequently in patients with poor control of the upper airway, during periods of poor synchronization of respiratory muscle contraction with the ventilator, and during sleep when upper airway tone is reduced. It has been recommended that patients undergoing nighttime negative pressure ventilation have sleep studies to evaluate possible obstructive events. Patients with poor control of upper airway musculature or obstructive sleep apnea should not be treated with any negative pressure device because this may result in occlusion of the airway and significant risk of hypercapnia and hemoglobin desaturation.[29]

Positive pressure ventilators
Positive pressure ventilators function by applying positive pressure to the airways, thus promoting the movement of air into the lungs. Exhalation of gases occurs passively with relaxation of the chest wall and lung. Positive pressure ventilation can be delivered to those requiring chronic ventilation in several ways – "invasively" via an indwelling tracheostomy and "noninvasively" via a mask interface.

Invasive PPV using an indwelling tracheostomy has been used successfully in several large series.[35,89,90] The development of convenient, portable positive pressure generators has made this form of ventilation practical. Benefits of this type of ventilator support include complete control of the machine-delivered tidal gas volume and ease of access to the central airways for suctioning of secretions. In addition, treatment during episodes of acute respiratory failure requires no change in the method of ventilation.

Unfortunately, several serious complications from long-term PPV have been cited. Damage to the trachea from the indwelling tube, including tracheal necrosis, stenosis, and hemorrhage, and tracheoesophageal fistulae have been reported.[91] However, the development of low-pressure, high-volume cuffed plastic tracheostomy tubes has reduced the incidence of these complications. Food aspiration and swallowing problems can also occur from interference with the normal swallowing mechanism. An increased risk of airway colonization with bacteria and lower respiratory tract infections has also been noted. The use of a tracheostomy tube requires supplemental humidification, an additional daily respiratory care task. Finally, social interactions and patient psychologic well-being may be impaired by the inability to speak, which is associated with the tracheostomy tube. Several devices and techniques have been designed to allow speech and communication while the patient is on the ventilator, including one-way valves that allow gas to pass through the vocal cords during exhalation (Passy-Muir Valve; Passy-Muir, Irvine, CA) and the "Trach-Talk" tracheostomy tube (Portex, Keene, NH), which has a channel to direct compressed air through the vocal cords. Unfortunately, not all individuals can use these devices.

Noninvasive delivery of PPV was first used during the polio epidemics of the 1950s to allow patients time out of the iron lung. More recently, there has been significant renewed interest in this technique. There are a variety of available mask interfaces including mouthpiece, nasal mask, nasal pillows, and full face mask (**Fig. 5**).

When leakage of air occurs, there may be oxyhemoglobin desaturation, elevation of arterial CO_2, and associated symptoms. In this situation, the use of a chin strap or full oral-facial mask interface may be appropriate.[92]

It has been suggested that the use of noninvasive positive pressure devices be avoided in patients (1) with coexisting severe lung disease when secretions may be a problem; (2) who are obtunded or uncooperative; (3) when poor oropharyngeal muscle strength is present and secretions cannot be handled effectively; (4) who have uncontrolled seizure disorders; and (5) with orthopedic conditions that interfere with placement of the devices. These represent relative instead of absolute contraindications, and experienced practitioners and motivated patients may still be able to use NIV, even in these situations.

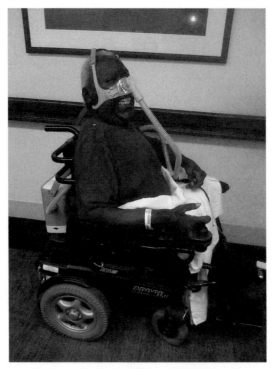

Fig. 5. Noninvasive ventilation with the Use of a nasal mask interface.

Noninvasive PPV has been used with excellent results in a wide range of patients. Patients who require only nocturnal ventilatory support may be particularly suitable candidates for this form of therapy. However, reports of long-term 24-hour NIV use have been published suggesting that need for full-time ventilator support does not always rule out the use of NIV.[93] In some cases, patients using invasive forms of ventilation have been switched effectively to noninvasive PPV, thus avoiding the problems of tracheostomy.[92]

Noninvasive PPV can be delivered with several different types of ventilators.[94,95] With one of these machines, the positive pressure delivered to the patient is high during inspiration and lower during expiration (bilevel positive pressure inspiration). The positive pressure gradient during inspiration results in delivery of a tidal volume to the patient. Exhalation still occurs passively and is terminated when the airway pressure returns to the lower expiratory level. Because the expiratory pressure is greater than atmospheric, the end-expiratory lung volume is increased. Newer technology provides automatic pressure adjustments for patients with progressive respiratory dysfunction, as commonly seen in patients with NMDs. One such technology guarantees a certain volume of air per minute using the average volume assured pressure support. This technology adapts to a patient's changing needs by calculating the change in pressure needed to achieve a preset target tidal volume and then slowly increases or decreases the IPAP pressure to meet this goal. No randomized studies comparing the efficacy of average volume assured pressure support to bilevel positive pressure inspiration have been completed; however, anecdotal evidence supports use of this assistive technology for 24-hour noninvasive ventilatory management in patients wishing to forgo invasive mechanical ventilation.

Ventilators Resulting in Passive Movement of the Diaphragm

Two types of "ventilators" that result in ventilation by acting on the abdominal contents to move the diaphragm passively are the "pneumobelt" and the rocking bed. The pneumobelt consists of an inflatable rubber bladder encased in a fabric corset that is strapped around the abdomen. A positive pressure generator attached to the pneumobelt will inflate the device, resulting in compression of abdominal contents, upward displacement of the diaphragm, and forced exhalation. When the bladder deflates, abdominal pressure is lowered and the diaphragm descends, resulting in a spontaneous inhalation of air into the patient's lungs. The patient must be seated at a 30° angle or greater from the horizontal device to function properly.[91,96] Therefore, daytime use is the most common application, and 24-hour use is not recommended.[91] The device may not be effective in obese patients, those with significant thoracic deformity, or those with a scaphoid abdomen.[97] Because the ventilator functions during exhalation, a significant benefit for some patients is louder and clearer speech. In addition, the use of the pneumobelt may result in more free time off other forms of ventilation. Some patients may even have had tracheostomies removed and learn to use glossopharyngeal breathing when the pneumobelt is not in use.

Another form of "ventilator" that uses gravitation-induced movement of the abdominal contents and diaphragm to achieve ventilation is the "rocking bed." This device originally was used on patients with poliomyelitis in the early 1950s.[98] It consists of a motorized bed that moves through an area of about 45° above the horizontal, 12 to 15 times per minute. As the head of the bed tilts downward, gravity forces the abdominal contents and diaphragm upward into the chest, resulting in forced exhalation. As the head of the bed is tilted upward, the diaphragm and abdominal contents shift downward, with resulting inhalation of air. The rocking bed is most appropriate for patients who require ventilator assistance less than 24 hours per day who are able to use it at night.

Diaphragm Pacing

Electric stimulation of the diaphragm by pacing with implanted electrodes with either direct phrenic nerve stimulation with nerve cuff electrodes (Avery Biomedical Devices, Commack, New York) or intramuscular electrodes (Cleveland Clinic System, Cleveland, Ohio) is a technique available to patients with intact phrenic nerves and diaphragm muscle adequate to sustain ventilation when stimulated (**Fig. 6**). It is used most often in patients with central alveolar hypoventilation and in patients with paralysis of the respiratory muscles secondary to high (C1-C2) cervical cord injuries[99] or congenital central hypoventilation syndrome.[100]

Diaphragm pacing with intramuscular stimulation of phrenic nerve motor points has been used in ALS.[101,102] Unlike when using a pacer in the setting of spinal cord injury, in ALS the pacer is used as therapy instead of a form of ventilator support. Intermittent use of the pacer throughout the day assists in fortifying muscle function[103] and extending muscle life in the setting of ALS.[104] The use of the device has been shown to prolong life in patients with ALS, and on this basis, the Food and Drug Administration has approved this therapy. Given the small size of the study submitted to the Food and Drug Administration, other studies have recently been undertaken to better characterize the ultimate impact and best use of this device in ALS.[105] Diaphragm pacing is not indicated in respiratory muscle dysfunction because of lower motor neuron lesions involving the phrenic nerve or muscular dystrophy involving the diaphragm. Before considering diaphragm pacing in either ALS or spinal cord injury, phrenic nerve conduction studies should be performed to ensure adequate function.

The Avery diaphragm pacing device itself consists of 4 parts: 1 or 2 phrenic nerve electrodes, a radiofrequency receiver attached to the electrodes, an external coil or antenna, and an external radiofrequency transmitter that can be programmed with regard to frequency of electrical stimulation and duration of stimulation. The major

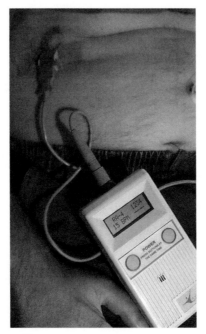

Fig. 6. Diaphragm pacing unit.

advantage of this system is the small, lightweight nature of the equipment, which leaves the patient less encumbered compared with standard ventilator techniques. The procedure requires operative implantation of the electrodes and receiver and is relatively expensive. In addition, upper airway obstruction during diaphragm contraction may be encountered, necessitating placement of a tracheostomy, and there is risk of infection of the implanted electrodes.

Adjunctive Respiratory Aids for the Patient With NMD

Mechanical ventilatory support as described earlier assists the patient's inspiratory muscles to maintain ventilation with normal CO_2 levels. However, hypoventilation represents only one of the respiratory problems encountered by patients with NMD. *Expiratory muscle function* is also frequently impaired, which leads to problems with effective cough that lead to frequent respiratory infections, pneumonia, and even death. Respiratory infection is one of the leading causes of death for the patient with NMD. A cough expiratory flow rate of at least 270 L/min has been suggested as the minimum flow rate necessary to produce an effective cough.[68] The patient with NMD frequently will need assistance to generate these flows.

Several approaches are available to increase cough expiratory flows in patients with NMD. Manually assisted coughing is a method of applying a positive pressure to the abdomen, pleural space, and airway, leading to adequate cough expiratory flow rates. Several techniques allow an attendant to apply rapid abdominal thrusts that result in effective clearance of secretions.[26] Patients can assist the attendant by taking a maximal inspiration before the abdominal thrusts are applied. Glossophyaryngeal breathing ("frog breathing) can be used to augment maximal inspiration in patients who cannot generate adequate inspiratory effort.[106]

Patients with severe obesity or kyphoscoliosis may not tolerate assisted cough techniques and may require additional intervention to maintain airway hygiene and avoid pneumonia. One such method, available for more than 40 years, is the MIE (In-exsufflator, JH Emerson Co, Cambridge, MA). This device consists of an electric motor that generates positive and negative pressures of up to 50 cm of H_2O to the airways of patients who are unable to cough. The pressure is applied via a facemask, mouthpiece, or tracheostomy adapter connected to the flow generator. Insufflation is applied to the respiratory system during a 1- to 3-second period by exerting a positive pressure of between 10 and 50 cm of H_2O. A negative pressure of between 20 and 50 cm H_2O is then rapidly applied to the airway by reversing the flow and secretions are suctioned from the airway noninvasively. A direct comparison of airway clearance techniques has shown that no technique works for every patient in every disease state. Instead, individual trials are needed to assess the most effective therapy option for each patient.[107]

EFFECTIVENESS OF CHRONIC VENTILATION IN NMD

Benefits ascribed to the use of chronic mechanical ventilation in patients with NMD are numerous and include reduced Pa_{CO_2} and increased PaO_2, on-and-off ventilator, decreased symptoms of respiratory failure, improved quality of life, and reduced morbidity and mortality. It has been clear for some time that intermittent ventilation may ameliorate symptoms of respiratory failure, reduce Pa_{CO_2}, increase PaO_2 (even during periods off the ventilator), and prolong survival in patients with NMD. Nocturnal ventilation has become a widely accepted clinical practice, providing ventilatory assistance for patients while sleeping, and allowing them to breathe on their own during the day. Curran reported on the initial use of the nocturnal negative pressure ventilation in patients with late-stage DMD.[34] In patients who had symptoms of ventilatory failure and $Paco_2$ of 50 mm Hg or higher, nocturnal negative pressure ventilation using cuirass or tank ventilators significantly improved arterial $Paco_2$ values (60.8 mm Hg pretreatment to 45.5 mm Hg posttreatment) and $Paco_2$ values (59.3 mm Hg pretreatment and 74.6 mm Hg posttreatment). Since that time, several published studies have reported using nocturnal ventilation and have supported these findings.[29–31,34,35]

The mechanics by which intermittent nocturnal ventilation results in amelioration of respiratory failure have not been entirely elucidated but probably are multifactorial. During periods of mechanical ventilation, there is a significant reduction in diaphragm and accessory muscle electromyographic activity.[108,109] This reduction in electromyographic activity likely signifies a decrease in work performed and oxygen consumed by the respiratory muscles. Some authors have postulated that nighttime ventilation rests fatigued respiratory muscles, allowing improved daytime function.[110] The rest provided by this reduction in work load may reverse chronic respiratory muscle fatigue thought to be present in these patients, allowing improved daytime function. In one study daytime inspiratory muscle *endurance* was noted to increase from 7.1 ± 3.4 minutes to 14.8 ± 7.6 minutes 3 months after initiation of nighttime ventilation.[23] Results of studies evaluating improvement in muscle *strength* have been mixed, with some authors noting slight improvements and others noting no improvement.[29,110]

A second hypothesis explaining the improvement in daytime respiratory function with nocturnal ventilation is related to reversing the adverse effects of chronic NMD on respiratory system mechanics.[111] Improvements in lung compliance, increases in resting lung volumes, and a decrease in the work of breathing have been reported[34,50] in patients with NMD after PPV.[110,111] If these improvements were sustained throughout the day, they would constitute a reduced load on the respiratory muscles, which would ameliorate chronic fatigue. In addition, increases in end-expiratory lung volumes to more normal ranges would reduce atelectasis and improve oxygenation.

A third explanation involves the reversal of what has been referred to as "central fatigue" in which nighttime hypoventilation and hypoxemia are thought to lead to a blunting of central respiratory drive, resulting in "adaptive" daytime hypoventilation.[112] It has been postulated that nighttime ventilatory intervention results in a "resetting" of central control mechanisms with an increase in chemosensitivity and a reduction of the body bicarbonate pool.[23] Increases in $Paco_2$ would be met with a more appropriate response in minute ventilation. Data to support this hypothesis are not currently available. It is possible that all 3 of these mechanisms are involved in the improvement of arterial blood gas values and daytime function noted in patients treated with nocturnal ventilation.

In addition to improvement in arterial blood gases, other measures of physiologic function have been shown to improve with intermittent ventilation. Hoeppner and colleagues[111] showed increases in vital capacity, reduction in erythrocytosis, and improvement in right-sided heart failure following nighttime ventilation, with changes maintained during a mean follow-up period of 3.4 years.

For ethical reasons, no randomized controlled trial evaluating the effect on survival of intervention with mechanical ventilation has been performed in patients with NMD. It is clear in most progressive NMDs that once an elevation in $Paco_2$ and a decrease in $Paco_2$ are noted, cor pulmonale and death are inevitable within a short time. It is therefore accepted by most authors that mechanical ventilation in the home leads to improved survival in most patients.

The institution of home mechanical ventilation also has enabled patients to improve their quality of life. These patients need not be confined to the home and its nearby environs. It is possible, however, for some patients to lead fully productive lives. Those requiring only nocturnal ventilation can be fully employed or attend school full-time.[93,113,114] For those requiring 24-hour ventilator assistance, portable ventilators adaptable for carrying on specialized wheelchairs are available, allowing access to the community. Many patients receiving nocturnal ventilation will notice a dramatic improvement in daytime alertness and functional activities, and some may become active with minimal assistance.

COSTS OF MECHANICAL VENTILATION IN NMD

The costs of caring for patients who require prolonged mechanical ventilation can be enormous. This results from the impressive number of technologic devices required to maintain artificial respiration and the considerable requirements for attendant care. Davis and colleagues[115] studied the hospital costs of patients requiring mechanical ventilation for longer than 48 hours. In their study, the mean charge for these patients per hospitalization was approximately 8 times that for all other hospitalized patients. In patients who are unable to wean from the ventilator and require chronic care, costs can range up to *$66,000* per month.[116]

The cost for home mechanical ventilation varies depending on the type of ventilator required, the number of other respiratory therapy devices required, and the level of assistance for care required. In 1992, Bach and colleagues[116] reported their experience in 20 adult ventilator-assisted individuals who had lived in long-term hospital care settings and subsequently been moved to their homes for chronic care. In-hospital costs averaged $718.80 per patient day, whereas home care cost on average $235.13 per day. This decrease of 77% resulted in an annual yearly savings to the health care system of $176,137 per patient.

The most important determinant of cost for home care is the type of attendant engaged in personal care of ventilator-assisted individuals. In the patient with a tracheostomy that requires suction, some states have required the use of licensed nursing. A study published in 1996, by Sevick and colleagues[117] examined the varying cost of home ventilator care dependent on the type of attendant providing the care. Using licensed practical nurse rates for private duty care, the average total cost of care was estimated to be $7642 per month. Using registered nurse rates for private duty care, the average total cost of home care was estimated to be $8596 per month, increasing the cost of home care significantly. Several groups have endorsed the use of properly trained nonlicensed attendants in the home care of ventilator-assisted individuals.[93,116,118,119] To the extent that family members can be trained to perform patient care activities, costs may be reduced even further. Accordingly, careful training of family members before patient discharge from the acute care setting is important. Family members frequently can provide excellent attendant care, reducing the need for 24-hour care by trained individuals. This can reduce costs to the health care system, although the financial burden in the form of loss of potential wages for family members has not been studied in detail. Once mechanical ventilation is instituted, it has been reported to decrease hospitalization in patients with NMD.[120]

SUMMARY

The clinician working with patients with NMD should be aware of the effects of muscle weakness on the respiratory system. Symptoms may present insidiously and can result in progressive loss of function, respiratory failure, and even death. Several techniques, including several forms of mechanical ventilation and physical aids to assist airway hygiene, are available and are effective in improving symptoms and survival in appropriately selected patients with NMD.

REFERENCES

1. Gilroy J, Cahalan JL, Berman R, et al. Cardiac and pulmonary complications in Duchenne's progressive muscular dystrophy. Circulation 1963;27:484–93.
2. Miller RG, Jackson CE, Kasarskis EJ, et al. Practice parameter update: the care of the patient with amyotrophic lateral sclerosis: drug, nutritional, and respiratory therapies (an evidence-based review): report of the Quality Standards Subcommittee of the American Academy of Neurology. Neurology 2009;73:1218–26.
3. Bushby K, Finkel R, Birnkrant DJ, et al. Diagnosis and management of Duchenne muscular dystrophy, part 2: implementation of multidisciplinary care. Lancet Neurol 2010;9(2):177–89.
4. Mehta S. Neuromuscular disease causing acute respiratory failure. Respir Care 2006;51(9):1016–21 [discussion: 1021–3].
5. Braun NMT, Aurora NS, Rochester DF. Respiratory muscle and pulmonary function in poliomyositis and other proximal myopathies. Thorax 1983;38:316–23.
6. Carratù P, Cassano A, Gadaleta F, et al. Association between low sniff nasal-inspiratory pressure (SNIP) and sleep disordered breathing in amyotrophic lateral sclerosis: Preliminary results. Amyotroph Lateral Scler 2011;12(6):458–63.
7. Morgan RK, McNally S, Alexander M, et al. Use of Sniff nasal- inspiratory force to predict survival in amyotrophic lateral sclerosis. Am J Respir Crit Care Med 2005;171:269–74.
8. Lechtzin N, Wiener CM, Shade DM, et al. Spirometry in the supine position improves the detection of diaphragmatic weakness in patients with amyotrophic lateral sclerosis. Chest 2002;121(2):436–42.
9. Schmidt EP, Drachman DB, Wiener CM, et al. Pulmonary predictors of survival in amyotrophic lateral sclerosis: use in clinical trial design. Muscle Nerve 2006; 33(1):127–32.
10. Katz S, Gaboury I, Keilty K, et al. Nocturnal hypoventilation: predictors and outcomes in childhood progressive neuromuscular disease. Arch Dis Child 2010;95:998–1003.
11. Hukins CA, Hillman DR. Daytime predictors of sleep hypoventilation in Duchenne muscular dystrophy. Am J Respir Crit Care Med 2000;161:166–70.
12. Lechtzin N, Scott Y, Busse A, et al. Early use of non-invasive ventilation prolongs survival in subjects with ALS. Amyotroph Lateral Scler 2007;8(3):185–8.
13. Bach J, Saporito L. Criteria for extubation and tracheostomy tube removal for patients with ventilatory failure. A different approach to weaning. Chest 1996; 110(6):1566–71.
14. Bergofsky EH. Respiratory failure in disorders of the thoracic cage. Am Rev Respir Dis 1979;119:643–69.
15. Estenne M, Heilporn A, Delhez L, et al. Chest wall stiffness in patients with chronic respiratory muscle weakness. Am Rev Respir Dis 1983;128(6):1002–7.
16. McCool FD, Mayewski RF, Shayne DS, et al. Intermittent positive pressure breathing in patients with respiratory muscle weakness. Alterations in total respiratory system compliance. Chest 1986;90(4):546–52.
17. Kirk V. Pulmonary complications of neuromuscular disease. Paediatr Respir Rev 2006;7(Suppl 1):S232–4.
18. Wazeka AN, DiMaio MF, Boachie-Adjei O. Outcome of pediatric patients with severe restrictive lung disease following reconstructive spine surgery. Spine 2004;29:528–35.
19. Barois A. Respiratory problems in severe scoliosis. Bull Acad Natl Med 1999; 183:721–30.

20. Muirhead A. The assessment of lung function in children with scoliosis. J Bone Joint Surg Am 1985;67:699–702.
21. Annane D, Quera-Salva MA, Lofaso F, et al. Mechanisms underlying effects of nocturnal ventilation on daytime blood gases in neuromuscular diseases. Eur Respir J 1999;13:157–62.
22. Perrin C, Unterborn J, D'Ambrosia C, et al. Pulmonary complications of chronic neuromuscular diseases and their management. Muscle Nerve 2004;29:5–27.
23. Goldstein RS, Molotiu N, Skrastins R, et al. Reversal of sleep-induced hypoventilation and chronic respiratory failure by nocturnal negative pressure ventilation in patients with restrictive ventilatory impairment. Am Rev Respir Dis 1987;135: 1049–55.
24. Ragette R, Mellies U, Schwake C, et al. Patterns and predictors of sleep disordered breathing in primary myopathies. Thorax 2002;57:724–8.
25. Guilleminault C, Kurland G, Winkle R, et al. Severe kyphoscoliosis, breathing, and sleep: the "Quasimodo" syndrome during sleep. Chest 1981;79(6):626–30.
26. Mezon BL, West P, Israels J, et al. Sleep breathing abnormalities in kyphoscoliosis. Am Rev Respir Dis 1980;122:617–20.
27. Bach JR. Pulmonary rehabilitation. The obstructive and paralytic conditions. Philadelphia: Hanley & Belfus; 1995. p. 303–30.
28. Phillipson EA. Control of breathing during sleep. Am Rev Respir Dis 1978;118: 909–39.
29. Bach JR, Alba AS, Saporito LR. Intermittent positive pressure ventilation via the mouth as an alternative to tracheostomy for 257 ventilator users. Chest 1993; 103:174–82.
30. Ellis ER, Grunstein R, Chan S, et al. Noninvaasive ventilatory support during sleep improves respiratory failure in kyphoscoliosis. Chest 1988;94:811–5.
31. Gay PC, Patel AM, Viggiano RW, et al. Nocturnal nasal ventilation for treatment of patients with hypercapnic respiratory failure. Mayo Clin Proc 1991;66:695–703.
32. Heckmatt JZ, Loh L, Dubowitz V. Night-time nasal ventilation in neuromuscular disease. Lancet 1990;335:579–82.
33. Kerby GR, Mayer LS, Pingleton SK. Nocturnal positive pressure ventilation via nasal mask. Am Rev Respir Dis 1987;135:738–40.
34. Curran FJ. Night ventilation by body respirators for patients in chronic respiratory failure due to late stage. Duchenne muscular dystrophy. Arch Phys Med Rehabil 1981;62:270–4.
35. Ellis ER, Bye PT, Bruderer JW, et al. Treatment of respiratory failure during sleep in patients with neuromuscular disease. Am Rev Respir Dis 1987;135:148–52.
36. Splaingard ML, Frates RC Jr, Harrison GM, et al. Home positive-pressure ventilation. Twenty years' experience. Chest 1983;84(4):376–92.
37. Melo J, Homma A, Iturriaga E, et al. Pulmonary evaluation and prevalence of noninvasive ventilation in patients with amyotrophic lateral sclerosis: a multicenter survey and proposal of a pulmonary protocol. J Neurol Sci 1999;169:114–7.
38. Lechtzin N, Wiener CM, Clawson L, et al. Use of noninvasive ventilation in patients with amyotrophic lateral sclerosis. Amyotroph Lateral Scler Other Motor Neuron Disord 2004;5(1):9–15.
39. Centers for Medicare & Medicaid Services, "LCD for Respiratory Assist Devices (L11504, L5023, L11493), " U.S. Department of Health and Human Services, (revision effective date 2/4/2011).
40. Finder JD, Birnkrant D, Carl J, et al. Respiratory care of the patient with Duchenne muscular dystrophy: ATS consensus statement. Am J Respir Crit Care Med 2004;170:456–65.

41. Phillips MF, Quinlivan CM, Edwards RH, et al. Changes in spirometry over time as a prognostic marker in patients with Duchenne muscular dystrophy. Am J Respir Crit Care Med 2001;164:2191–4.

42. Eagle M, Baudouin SV, Chandler C, et al. Survival in Duchenne muscular dystrophy: improvements in life expectancy since 1967 and the impact of home nocturnal ventilation. Neuromuscul Disord 2002;12:926–9.

43. Gomez-Merino E, Bach JR. Duchenne muscular dystrophy: prolongation of life by noninvasive ventilation and mechanically assisted coughing. Am J Phys Med Rehabil 2002;81:411–5.

44. Dohna-Schwake C, Ragette R, Teschler H, et al. Predictors of severe chest infections in pediatric neuromuscular disorders. Neuromuscul Disord 2006;16:325–8.

45. Bianchi C, Baiardi P. Cough peak flows: standard values for children and adolescents. Am J Phys Med Rehabil 2008;87:461–7.

46. Kang SW, Bach JR. Maximum insufflation capacity: vital capacity and cough flows in neuromuscular disease. Am J Phys Med Rehabil 2000;79:222–7.

47. Daftary AS, Crisanti M, Kalra M, et al. Effect of long-term steroids on cough efficiency and respiratory muscle strength in patients with Duchenne muscular dystrophy. Pediatrics 2007;117:e320–4.

48. Gauld LM, Boynton A. Relationship between peak cough flow and spirometry in Duchenne muscular dystrophy. Pediatr Pulmonol 2005;39:457–60.

49. Suarez AA, Pessolano FA, Monteiro SG, et al. Peak flow and peak cough flow in the evaluation of expiratory muscle weakness and bulbar impairment in patients with neuromuscular disease. Am J Phys Med Rehabil 2002;81:506–11.

50. Szeinberg A, Tabachnik E, Rashed N, et al. Cough capacity in patients with muscular dystrophy. Chest 1988;94:1232–5.

51. Smith PE, Calverley PM, Edwards RH. Hypoxemia during sleep in Duchenne muscular dystrophy. Am Rev Respir Dis 1988;137:884–8.

52. Phillips MF, Smith PE, Carroll N, et al. Nocturnal oxygenation and prognosis in Duchenne muscular dystrophy. Am J Respir Crit Care Med 1999;160:198–202.

53. Khan Y, Heckmatt JZ. Obstructive apnoeas in Duchenne muscular dystrophy. Thorax 1994;49:157–61.

54. Barbe F, Quera-Salva MA, McCann C, et al. Sleep-related respiratory disturbances in patients with Duchenne muscular dystrophy. Eur Respir J 1994;7:1403–8.

55. Uliel S, Tauman R, Greenfeld M, et al. Normal polysomnographic respiratory values in children and adolescents. Chest 2004;125:872–8.

56. Toussaint M, Steens M, Soudon P. Lung function accurately predicts hypercapnia in patients with Duchenne muscular dystrophy. Chest 2007;131:368–75.

57. Culebras A. Sleep-disordered breathing in neuromuscular disease. Sleep Med Clin 2008;3:377–86.

58. Eagle M, Bourke J, Bullock R, et al. Managing Duchenne muscular dystrophy—the additive effect of spinal surgery and home nocturnal ventilation in improving survival. Neuromuscul Disord 2007;17:470–5.

59. Ward S, Chatwin M, Heather S, et al. Randomised controlled trial of non-invasive ventilation (NIV) for nocturnal hypoventilation in neuromuscular and chest wall disease patients with daytime normocapnia. Thorax 2005;60:1019–24.

60. Bach JR, Alba AS. Management of chronic alveolar hypoventilation by nasal ventilation. Chest 1990;97:52–7.

61. Mellies U, Ragette R, Dohna Schwake C, et al. Long-term noninvasive ventilation in children and adolescents with neuromuscular disorders. Eur Respir J 2003;22:631–6.

62. Simonds AK, Muntoni F, Heather S, et al. Impact of nasal ventilation on survival in hypercapnic Duchenne muscular dystrophy. Thorax 1998;53:949–52.
63. Piastra M, Antonelli M, Caresta E, et al. Noninvasive ventilation in childhood acute neuromuscular respiratory failure. Respiration 2006;73:791–8.
64. Niranjan V, Bach JR. Noninvasive management of pediatric neuromuscular respiratory failure. Crit Care Med 1998;26:2061–5.
65. Bach JR, Bianchi C, Vidigal-Lopes M, et al. Lung inflation by glossopharyngeal breathing and air stacking in Duchenne muscular dystrophy. Am J Phys Med Rehabil 2007;86:295–300.
66. Bach JR, Kang SW. Disorders of ventilation: weakness, stiffness and mobilization. Chest 2000;117:301–3.
67. Misuri G, Lanini B, Gigliotti F, et al. Mechanism of CO2 retention in patients with neuromuscular disease. Chest 2000;117:447–53.
68. Tzeng AC, Bach JR. Prevention of pulmonary morbidity for patients with neuromuscular disease. Chest 2000;118:1390–6.
69. Dohna-Schwake C, Ragette R, Teschler H, et al. IPPB-assisted coughing in neuromuscular disorders. Pediatr Pulmonol 2006;41:551–7.
70. Miske LJ, Hickey EM, Kolb SM, et al. Use of the mechanical in-exsufflator in pediatric patients with neuromuscular disease and impaired cough. Chest 2004;125:1406–12.
71. Boitano JL. Management of airway clearance in neuromusculardisease. Respir Care 2006;51:913–22.
72. Fauroux B, Guillemot N, Aubertin G, et al. Physiological benefits of mechanical insufflation-exsufflation in children with neuromuscular diseases. Chest 2008; 133:161–8.
73. Chatwin M, Ross E, Hart N, et al. Cough augmentation with mechanical insufflation/exsufflation in patients with neuromuscular weakness. Eur Respir J 2003;21: 502–8.
74. Winck JC, Goncalves MR, Lourenco C, et al. Effects of mechanical insufflation-exsufflation on respiratory parameters for patients with chronic airway secretion encumbrance. Chest 2004;126:774–80.
75. Homnick DN. Mechanical insufflation-exsufflation for airway mucus clearance. Respir Care 2007;52:1296–305.
76. Bushby K, Finkel R, Birnkrant DJ, et al, for the DMD Care Considerations Working Group, Centers for Disease Control. Diagnosis and management of Duchenne muscular dystrophy, part 1: diagnosis, and pharmacological and psychosocial management. Lancet Neurol 2010;9(1):77–93.
77. Wang CH, Finkel RS, Bertini ES, et al, Participants of the International Conference on SMA Standard of Care. Consensus statement for standard of care in spinal muscular atrophy. J Child Neurol 2007;22(8):1027–49.
78. Schroth MK. Atrophy special considerations in the respiratory management of spinal muscular. Pediatrics 2009;123:S245.
79. Wang CH, Bonnemann CG, Rutkowski A, et al, International Standard of Care Committee for Congenital Muscular Dystrophy. Consensus statement on standard of care for congenital muscular dystrophies. J Child Neurol 2010;25(12):1559–81.
80. Yemen TA, McClain C. Muscular dystrophy, anesthesia and the safety of inhalational agents revisited, again. Paediatr Anaesth 2006;16:105–8.
81. Birnkrant DJ, Panitch HB, Benditt JO, et al. American College of Chest Physicians consensus statement on the respiratory and related management of patients with Duchenne muscular dystrophy undergoing anesthesia or sedation. Chest 2007;132:1977–86.

82. Bach JR, Sabharwal S. High pulmonary risk scoliosis surgery: role of noninvasive ventilation and related techniques. J Spinal Disord Tech 2005;18:527–30.

83. Lumbierres M, Prats E, Farrero E, et al. Noninvasive positive pressure ventilation prevents postoperative pulmonary complications in chronic ventilator users. Respir Med 2007;101:62–8.

84. Drinker P, Shaw LA. An apparatus for the prolonged administration of artificial respiration. J Clin Invest 1929;7:247–99.

85. Corrado A, Gorini M. Negative-pressure ventilation is there still a role. Eur Respir J 2002;20:187–97.

86. Collier CR, Affeldt JE. Ventilatory efficiency of the cuirass respirator in totally paralyzed chronic poliomyelitis patients. J Appl Physiol 1954;6:531–8.

87. Fink JB, Mahlmeister MJ. High-frequency oscillation of the airway and chest wall. Respir Care 2002;47(7):797–807.

88. Scharf SM, Feldman NT, Goldman MD, et al. Vocal cord closure. A cause of upper airway obstruction during controlled ventilation. Am Rev Respir Dis 1978;117(2):391–7.

89. Make BJ. Long-term management of ventilator-assisted individuals: the Boston University experience. Respir Care 1986;31:303–10.

90. Burr BH, Guyer B, Todres ID, et al. Home care for children on respirators. N Engl J Med 1983;309(21):1319–23.

91. Bach JR, Alba AS. Intermittent abdominal pressure ventilator in a regimen of noninvasive ventilatory support. Chest 1991;99:630–6.

92. Bach JR. Ventilatory support alternatives to tracheostomy and intubation: current status of the application of this technology. Conn Med 1991;55:323–9.

93. Bennditt JO. Full-time noninvasive ventilation: possible and desirable. Respir Care 2006;51(9):1005–12.

94. Strumpf DA, Carlisle CC, Millman RP, et al. An evaluation of the respironics BiPAP bilevel CPAP device for delivery of assisted ventilation. Respir Care 1990;35:415–22.

95. Waldhorn RE. Nocturnal nasal intermittent positive pressure ventilation with bilevel positive airway pressure (BiPAP) in respiratory failure. Chest 1991;101:516–21.

96. Adamson JP, Lewis L, Stein JD. Application of abdominal pressure for artificial respiration. JAMA 1959;169(14):1613–7.

97. Hill NS. Clinical application of body ventilators. Chest 1986;90:897–905.

98. Plum F, Whedon DA. The rapid-rocking bed: its effect on the ventilation of poliomyelitis patients with respiratory paralysis. N Engl J Med 1956;245:235–41.

99. Glenn WW, Hogan JF, Loke JS, et al. Ventilatory support by pacing of the conditioned diaphragm in quadriplegia. N Engl J Med 1984;310(18):1150–5.

100. Chen ML, Tablizo MA, Kun S, et al. Diaphragm pacers as a treatment for congenital central hypoventilation syndrome. Expert Rev Med Devices 2005; 2(5):577–85.

101. Onders RP, Elmo M, Khansarinia S, et al. Complete worldwide operative experience in laparoscopic diaphragm pacing: results and differences in spinal cord injured patients and amyotrophic lateral sclerosis patients. Surg Endosc 2009; 23(7):1433–40.

102. Onders RP, Carlin AM, Elmo M, et al. Amyotrophic lateral sclerosis: the Midwestern surgical experience with the diaphragm pacing stimulation system shows that general anesthesia can be safely performed. Am J Surg 2009;197(3): 386–90.

103. Costa D, Cancelliero KM, Campos GE, et al. Changes in types of muscle fibers induced by transcutaneous electrical stimulation of the diaphragm of rats. Braz J Med Biol Res 2008;41:809–11.
104. Onders RP. Non-Invasive Ventilation (NIV) and Diaphragm Pacing (DP): DP augments and improves the effectiveness of NIV in ALS/MND leading to an improved survival. Amyotroph Lateral Scler 2010;11:137.
105. Available at: http://www.clinicaltrials.gov/ct2/show/NCT01583088?term=als+and+pacing&rank=2. Accessed September 27, 2012
106. Bach JR, Alba AS, Bodofsky E, et al. Glossopharyngeal breathing and noninvasive aids in the management of post-polio respiratory insufficiency. Birth Defects Orig Artic Ser 1987;23:99–113.
107. Senet C, Golmard JL, Salachas F, et al. A comparison of assisted cough techniques in stable patients with severe respiratory insufficiency due to amyotrophic lateral sclerosis. Amyotroph Lateral Scler 2011;12:26–32.
108. Marino W, Braun NM. Reversal of the clinical sequelae of respiratory failure with nasal positive pressure ventilation. Am Rev Respir Dis 1982;125:185.
109. Sinha R, Bergofsky EH. Prolonged alteration of lung mechanics in kyphoscoliosis by positive pressure hyperinflation. Am Rev Respir Dis 1972;106:47–57.
110. Rochester DF, Braun NT, Lane S. Diaphragmatic energy expenditure in chronic respiratory failure. Am J Med 1977;63:223–32.
111. Hoeppner VH, Cockcroft DW, Dosman JA, et al. Night-time ventilation improves respiratory failure to secondary kyphoscoliosis. Am Rev Respir Dis 1984;129:240–3.
112. Roussos C. Function and fatigue of respiratory muscles. Chest 1985;88:1245–325.
113. Harrison GM, Mitchell MB. The medical and social outcome of 200 respirator and former respirator patients on home care. Arch Phys Med Rehabil 1961;42:590–8.
114. Make BJ, Gilmartin ME. Mechanical ventilation in the home. Crit Care Clin 1990;6:785–96.
115. Davis H, LeFrak SS, Miller D, et al. Prolonged mechanically assisted ventilation. An analysis of outcome and changes. JAMA 1980;243:43–5.
116. Bach JR, Intinola BA, Alba AS, et al. The ventilator-assisted individual. Cost analysis of institutionalization vs. rehabilitation and in-home management. Chest 1992;101:26–9.
117. Sevick MA, Kamlet MS, Hoffman LA, et al. Economic cost of home-based care for ventilator-assisted individuals: a preliminary report. Chest 1996;109(6):1597–606.
118. Goldberg A. Home care for life-supported persons – Is a national approach the answer? Chest 1986;90:744–8.
119. Goldberg AI, Faure EA, Vaughn CJ, et al. Home care for life-supported persons: an approach to program development. J Pediatr 1984;104:785–95.
120. Fischer DA, Prentice WS. Feasibility of home care for certain respiratory-dependent restrictive or obstructive lung disease patients. Chest 1982;82(6):739–43.

Cardiac Management in Neuromuscular Diseases

Hugh D. Allen, MD[a,b,c,d,*], Philip T. Thrush, MD[c],
Timothy M. Hoffman, MD[a,c], Kevin M. Flanigan, MD[a,b,e],
Jerry R. Mendell, MD[a,b,e]

KEYWORDS

- Duchenne muscular dystrophy • Becker muscular dystrophy
- Myotonic muscular dystrophy • Emery-Dreifuss muscular dystrophy
- Limb-girdle muscular dystrophy

KEY POINTS

- Various cardiac manifestations are seen in different types of muscular dystrophy, including cardiomyopathy and disturbances of conduction.
- Treatment strategies are evolving, with afterload reduction largely replacing use of digoxin in patients with cardiomyopathy with decreased ejection fraction.
- Careful genetic analysis allows proper classification of the various muscular dystrophies, resulting in proper diagnostic and treatment choices.

INTRODUCTION

This article addresses the present concepts regarding treatment of the more common neuromuscular diseases in children and young adults. These evolving strategies will likely be refined over time. Some are surrounded with debate, and differences are discussed. Treatment is predicated on accurate diagnosis, particularly genetic diagnosis, which is detailed in other articles in this issue. Cardiac diagnostic methods are briefly discussed. For more detail, the reader is referred to the chapter entitled "The Heart in the Muscular Dystrophies" in *Moss and Adams' Heart Disease in Infants, Children, and Adolescents: Including the Fetus and Young Adult*.[1,2]

[a] The Ohio State University College of Medicine, Columbus, OH, USA; [b] Center for Gene Therapy, Research Institute, Nationwide Children's Hospital, 700 Children's Drive, Columbus, OH 43205, USA; [c] The Heart Center, Nationwide Children's Hospital, 700 Children's Drive, Columbus, OH 43205, USA; [d] Baylor College of Medicine, Texas Children's Hospital Heart Center, 6621 Fannin street, Houston, TX 77030, USA; [e] Wellstone Muscular Dystrophy Cooperative Research Center, Rochester, NY, USA
* Corresponding author. Baylor College of Medicine, Texas Children's Hospital Heart Center, 6621 Fannin street, Houston, TX 77030
E-mail address: hdallen@texaschildrens.org

Phys Med Rehabil Clin N Am 23 (2012) 855–868
http://dx.doi.org/10.1016/j.pmr.2012.08.001
1047-9651/12/$ – see front matter © 2012 Elsevier Inc. All rights reserved.

CARDIAC DIAGNOSTIC METHODS

Common methods for cardiac evaluation include electrocardiography, Holter monitoring, Doppler echocardiography, and MRI. These modalities are discussed as they apply to the various neuromuscular diseases.

Electrocardiography

The electrocardiogram shows heart rhythm, rate, axis in the frontal plane, and changes in voltages interpreted as patterns of hypertrophy.

Holter Monitoring

Holter monitoring shows the heart rate patterns over a 24- or 48-hour time span. It can also reveal the presence of arrhythmias and ST-T wave abnormalities.

Cardiac Ultrasound

Doppler echocardiography shows cardiac anatomy and patterns of blood flow, which is especially important for evaluating left ventricular (LV) function. Areas of akinesis (lack of motion) or dyskinesis (abnormal motion) can be seen. LV remodeling, or rounding of the diseased ventricle, found with cardiomyopathy can be measured through comparing LV diastolic dimension and LV length (sphericity index). Systolic function can be measured through shortening fraction (LV end-diastolic dimension-LV end-systolic dimension vs LV end-diastolic dimension) and ejection fraction (LV systolic area vs LV diastolic area) (**Figs. 1** and **2**). Diastolic function can be assessed through measuring the LV diastolic dimension, relationship of mitral inflow velocities (E wave/A wave ratio), and tissue Doppler. Systolic and diastolic time intervals also reflect cardiomyopathy. The presence of aortic regurgitation and/or mitral regurgitation also can reflect LV dysfunction. Tricuspid and pulmonary regurgitation jet quantification can be used to predict pulmonary arterial pressures. With experience and perseverance, adequate imaging can be obtained in most patients with muscular dystrophy.

MRI

MRI allows superior anatomic definition and functional analysis compared with echocardiography but is more expensive and can cause claustrophobic reactions. Patients younger than 10 years usually require anesthesia. Scheduling MRI testing can be a problem because of limitations in availability. Furthermore, the presence of metallic

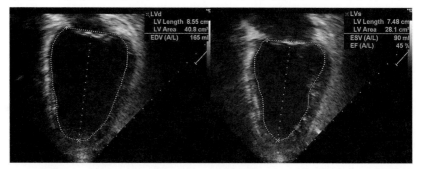

Fig. 1. Duchenne muscular dystrophy with cardiomyopathy. Echocardiogram, apex view, showing tracing for calculation of ejection fraction. Note that the LV is dilated. EDV(A/L), end diastolic volume-area/length; EF, ejection fraction; ESV, end diastolic volume; LV, left ventricle; LVd, left ventricle diastole; LVs, LV systole.

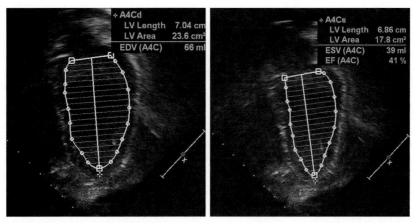

Fig. 2. Duchenne muscular dystrophy with cardiomyopathy. Echocardiogram, apex view, showing tracing for calculation of ejection fraction. The LV is not dilated. A4Cd = 4 chamber view, diastole; A4Cs, 4 chamber view, systolic; EDV(A/L), end diastolic volume-area/length; ESV, end diastolic volume; LV, left ventricle.

objects, such as pacemakers or rods used in scoliosis surgery, can interfere with imaging.

MUSCULAR DYSTROPHIES INVOLVING THE HEART
Dystrophinopathies

The 2 common dystrophinopathies are Duchenne muscular dystrophy (DMD) and Becker muscular dystrophy. According to clinical definitions of these X-linked disorders, patients who are ambulatory at 15 years of age have Becker muscular dystrophy. The genetic definition separates the 2 based on the *DMD* gene exon deletion: out-of-frame for Duchenne and in-frame for Becker. Furthermore, on muscle biopsy, little or no (<5%) dystrophin is seen in patients with DMD, whereas more is present in patients with Becker muscular dystrophy. Symptoms of heart failure are virtually absent in wheelchair-dependent patients with DMD, but ambulatory patients with Becker muscular dystrophy will have symptoms of shortness of breath and fatigue with ambulation.

DMD

History and physical examination
Patients with DMD are rarely symptomatic unless they are ambulatory. An apical S3 and S4 may be present in advanced cardiomyopathy. Additionally, a mitral regurgitation murmur may be audible. Patients with advanced disease may have signs of heart failure, including neck vein distention, sacral edema, peripheral edema, and hepatomegaly.

Pathology
Cardiac involvement in DMD is caused by fibrosis and scarring that proceeds from the epicardium to the endocardium, starting generally at the region behind the posterior mitral valve apparatus.[3–5] This scarring spreads downward progressively toward the apex and around the heart, ultimately leading to cardiomyopathy. The myopathy is not always dilated, because the scarred areas do not have expansile properties. This process has been confirmed in vivo by MRI studies.[6,7] A similar process is seen in Becker muscular dystrophy, and a recent study has shown that determining the exon deletion site has predictive value in estimating the timing of cardiomyopathy onset.[8]

Electrocardiography

The classic findings in DMD include a shortened PR interval, right ventricular hypertrophy (RVH), and Q waves in the inferolateral leads.[9–14] Previous literature suggested that Q waves in leads I and aVL were common and that RVH was proportional to the degree of myopathy, suggesting that LV fibrosis interfered with LV forces.[10–13] A large study showed that findings are present in approximately half of patients (43% short PR, 37% RVH, 34% Q wave in V5, V6)[14] (**Fig. 3**), with no relationship to the degree or presence of cardiomyopathy as defined by an echocardiography-derived ejection fraction of less than 55%. Furthermore, the presence of Q waves was more often seen in the inferolateral leads than the anterior leads.[14] An unpublished serial evaluation of R wave amplitudes in V1 showed no significant progression of that waveform over time in patients with cardiomyopathy of DMD (Thrush PT, Allen HD, unpublished data, 2012).

Holter monitoring

Several studies[15–18] have shown abnormally fast average heart rates in patients with DMD, regardless of the presence of cardiomyopathy. This condition is termed *disordered automaticity*, which is generally defined as an average heart rate exceeding 100 beats per minute in patients older than 12 years. It is attributed to a sympathetic imbalance. Older boys (and some younger ones) can have atrial and ventricular ectopy, heart block, and either atrial or ventricular tachydysrhythmias.[19,20]

Doppler echocardiography studies

Anatomically, LV posterior wall thinning can occasionally be appreciated, along with contractile and relaxation abnormalities. Using the parameters mentioned earlier, as the disease advances, areas of akinesis or dyskinesis can be seen, accompanied by some with LV dilation, decreased shortening fraction, rounding (remodeling) shown by a sphericity index approaching unity, and decreased ejection fraction. Diastolic

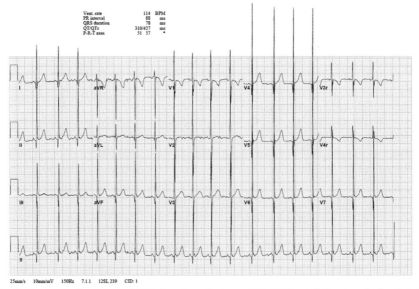

Fig. 3. Electrocardiogram in DMD showing shortened PR, RVH, and Q waves in leads II, III, aVF, V5, and V6 (inferolateral leads).

abnormalities can be seen with increasing mitral valve inflow Doppler E and A wave ratios and lateral and medial tissue Doppler ratios approaching unity.[21–30]

MRI studies
MRI can show the presence and distribution of myocardial fibrosis and offer a measurement of contractility and circumferential strain (**Fig. 4**). These findings precede the cardiomyopathy defined by an ejection fraction of less than 55% shown on echocardiographic studies.[6,7] Careful analysis of ejection fraction is also possible with MRI.

Laboratory analysis: biomarkers
Serum brain natriuretic peptide (BNP) and α-atrial natriuretic peptide (α-ANP) levels are elevated in the presence of LV dysfunction in adults and in some boys with DMD and advanced heart failure.[31,32]

Treatment of Cardiomyopathy in Dystrophinopathy

Timing of treatment initiation
Ideally, boys with DMD should be referred to a cardiologist for an initial evaluation at the time of diagnosis. Changes in the heart have been documented from an early age, with 53% of children aged 5 years and younger showing an abnormality on

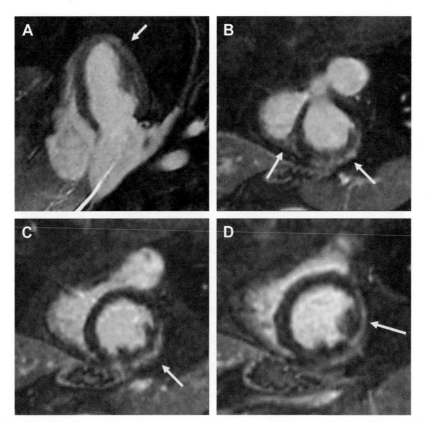

Fig. 4. MRI in patient with DMD. Note the whitened areas (*arrows*) reflecting fibrosis in the LV posterior wall.

electrocardiogram. Follow-up surveillance should continue every other year until the child begins to have symptoms or reaches the age of 10 years, when yearly follow-up should be initiated.

When to begin treating these patients with pharmacologic management is debated. Because these boys may not have symptoms, the standard has been to commence therapy if the echocardiography-derived ejection fraction is less than 55%.[29,33–37] This timing is parallel with that of treatment of other forms of cardiomyopathy. Some have initiated treatment if, in addition to the presence of echocardiographic abnormalities, biomarkers (α-ANP, BNP) are abnormal.[31,32]

Preventive treatment

Some centers advocate beginning treatment before echocardiographic abnormalities manifest, arguing that all of these boys have cardiomyopathy (raising the question, what is a cardiomyopathy?) regardless of the later-stage echocardiographic abnormalities. Duboc and colleagues[33,38] conducted a trial of placebo versus angiotensin-converting enzyme inhibitor (ACE-I) in boys with DMD who had normal ejection fraction on radioisotope analysis, with all boys placed on the ACE-I after 3 years. Although all patients showed progressive deterioration in function, no significant difference was seen between the groups in their ejection fractions over time, regardless of whether they were treated. More patients in the placebo group died than in the treated group at a 10-year follow-up. Because of the increased death rate (Kaplan-Meyer survival lower in the placebo group; $P = .13$), the investigators concluded that boys should be treated prophylactically after the age of 9.5 years. Although the causes of deaths were not detailed, the study has resulted in many centers adopting a preventive treatment approach.

An important MRI study by Hor and colleagues[6] showed that boys with normal echocardiographic ejection fraction had fibrosis and decreased peak circumferential strain on MRI. Patients younger than 10 years showed abnormal strain, and older boys showed a further decline in strain, with abnormal ejection fraction appearing at a mean age of 15.8 years.

A mouse model of DMD[39] showed a protective effect of Aldactone in combination with an ACE-I on both skeletal and cardiac muscle. This effect may be from the anti-fibrotic effects of these medications (transforming growth factor β inhibition) in treated mice versus controls. Clinical trials are obviously needed before this may be potentially translatable to boys with DMD.

Drugs and treatments used in cardiomyopathy of DMD

In the past, standard treatment was with digoxin and diuretics; however, because of the arrhythmogenic potential of digoxin, it has largely fallen out of favor.

The standard treatment of cardiomyopathy in adults has been ACE-I, and several centers have used the same concept in boys with cardiomyopathy of DMD.[29,33–37] At the authors' center, an analysis of 42 boys[37] showed that the mean age of onset of cardiomyopathy was 14.1 years, with a range of 7 to 27.3 years. Use of ACE-I resulted in ejection fraction improvement from a mean of 44% to 52% ($P \leq .001$). Addition of, or initial use of, a β-blocker before ACE-I initiation (usually for disordered automaticity) did not change the result ($P = .947$).

Angiotensin receptor blocker treatment can be effective and is associated with less cough (a rare complication of ACE-I). Furthermore, at least in the *mdx* mouse, skeletal and cardiac muscle regeneration has been seen. Clinical studies are needed to determine whether this occurs in humans. One such Muscular Dystrophy Association–sponsored study is underway.

Whether eplerenone or aldactone (both aldosterone antagonists) is effective in treating cardiomyopathy or reducing skeletal muscle degeneration requires careful and prospective double-blinded clinical studies.

For severe heart failure, hospitalization and treatment with milrinone may be useful. One study[40] has advocated using intravenous milrinone as home therapy, but this is not without potential adverse events, and most centers reserve this treatment for the inpatient arena.

Idebenone (a benzoquinone with antioxidant properties) improves respiratory chain function and cellular energy production and was found to be beneficial in a trial[41] in patients with DMD. Improvement in pulmonary function was also seen. A larger trial is ongoing. Trials are also underway assessing the use of sildenafil and carvedilol.

Atrial and ventricular arrhythmias are treated as per standard. For disordered automaticity, β-blocker therapy is used. If ventricular tachydysrhythmias are present, sotalol (a class III antiarrhythmic) or flecainide (a class Ic antiarrhythmic) may be used.

Automatic implantable cardioverter defibrillator placement may be helpful in patients with ventricular tachydysrhythmias, and is also considered in patients with an ejection fraction less than 15%, similar to the approach used in adults with severe congestive heart failure.

Another observation has been that boys with DMD can have hyperkalemic or hyperthermic reactions to inhalant anesthetic agents or muscle relaxants, suggesting that these agents should be avoided during general anesthesia.[42,43]

Use of nocturnal bilevel positive airway pressure (BiPAP) for respiratory support also benefits boys with cardiomyopathy. Although BiPAP results in decreased preload, the primary benefit is secondary to decreased LV transmural pressure and, ultimately, decreased afterload. With advances in pulmonary and cardiac treatment, these patients, although lacking skeletal muscle function, now survive longer.

Some providers consider using destination therapy (eg, extracorporeal membrane oxygenation, acutely, or left ventricular–assist devices, which can be used over a long term) in patients with DMD with severe cardiomyopathy, using the survival argument, although the ethics of this approach can be debated. The same argument can be made for cardiac transplantation. The ultimate hope is that gene therapy may reverse or stop the disease. Whether the cardiac myocyte response to gene therapy will be the same as the skeletal muscle response remains to be seen.

BECKER MUSCULAR DYSTROPHY

Cardiomyopathy in patients with Becker muscular dystrophy is treated in much the same manner as in DMD (**Fig. 5**). However, in severe heart failure, because boys with Becker muscular dystrophy live longer and are often ambulatory, destination therapies and transplantation are viable options.

Female Carriers and Dystrophic Cardiomyopathy

Often cardiac disease is the only manifestation that the carrier experiences, with the risk for cardiomyopathy increasing with age. In a study of female carriers, no subjects showed signs of cardiomyopathy at ages younger than 16 years. However, as age increased from 16 to 50 years, the rate of cardiomyopathy increased from 6% to 16%. Current treatment recommendations include providing a baseline cardiac evaluation as a young adult, with follow-up occurring at least every 5 years thereafter. Every effort should be made to counsel the carrier on the benefits of cardiac risk reduction strategies, including smoking cessation, hypertension management, and maintenance of a healthy weight and normal cholesterol levels.

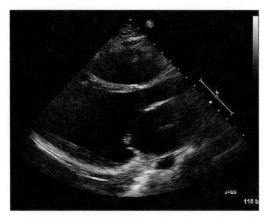

Fig. 5. Long axis view of dilated cardiomyopathy in Becker muscular dystrophy in a patient awaiting transplant. Ejection fraction was 18%.

MYOTONIC MUSCULAR DYSTROPHY

As discussed elsewhere in this issue, myotonic muscular dystrophy is the most common adult form of muscular dystrophy. More than one type of this disease exists.[43,44] The most common form, dystrophia myotonica type I (DM1), intensifies from generation to generation as a dominantly inherited disease, whereby repeats in the untranslated CTG region of the myotonic dystrophy protein kinase gene increase on chromosome 19. The repeat size often increases from generation to generation, referred to as "anticipation." Patients with DM1 can have conduction abnormalities.[45] The most severe form of the disease is congenital DM1, seen in some infants in whom the CTG repeat is markedly expanded. In almost all cases, the maternal parent has adult-onset DM1. Congenital DM1 can present with severe dilated cardiomyopathy, disturbances of rhythm, and death. A second form, DM2, has a different molecular defect, a CCTG repeat, in the zinc finger protein 9 gene on chromosome 3. Its cardiac manifestations are similar to those seen in adults with DM1.

Clinical Presentation of Myotonic Dystrophy

Patients commonly experience sleep and gastrointestinal disturbances before any muscle manifestations. Muscle weakness is noted in the face, neck, and limb muscles. Distal weakness is equal to or greater than proximal weakness. Patients will often develop early cataracts and can have baldness, diabetes, and infertility.[46]

The cardiac manifestations include conduction abnormalities, bradycardia, prolonged PR intervals, atrial fibrillation/flutter, atrioventricular block, prolongation of QRS and QTc intervals, ventricular tachycardia, and ventricular fibrillation. These findings typically worsen over time in approximately 75% of patients. Rarely, dilated cardiomyopathy will be present in adults with DM1 or DM2.[46–50]

Recent MRI studies have shown fatty infiltration of the right ventricle in patients with ventricular tachydysrhythmias.[51]

Treatment of Cardiac Problems Seen With Myotonic Dystrophy

Standard antiarrhythmic treatments should be tailored to the specific abnormality seen. Pacemaker placement can be lifesaving in patients with heart block.[52] Those with torsades de pointes, ventricular tachycardia, and/or ventricular fibrillation may require implantable cardioverter defibrillator placement. If cardiomyopathy is present, therapeutic regimens similar to those used in DMD and Becker muscular dystrophy may apply, including destination therapy and transplantation.

EMERY-DREIFUSS MUSCULAR DYSTROPHY

Two genetic forms of this disease are present; X-linked dominant forms and a recessive lamin A/C gene abnormality.[53–56] These patients have contractures in the elbow, Achilles tendon, posterior neck with later weakness in the upper arm, and peroneal muscles with later pectoral, knee, and hip extensor weakness.

Cardiac Manifestations

A progressive fatty and fibrotic infiltration of the atria occurs that ultimately results in both mechanical and conduction paralysis.[54–61] Electrocardiogram findings show progressive PR interval prolongation to atrioventricular block (**Fig. 6**). Patients may have atrial fibrillation/flutter, bradyarrhythmias, and tachyarrhythmias (**Fig. 7**). Cerebrovascular accidents can result from atrial clots breaking loose into the circulation. Some will have dilated cardiomyopathy.

Cardiac Treatment

Pacemaker therapy can be lifesaving; timing is a difficult issue, but erring on the side of aggressiveness is probably appropriate.[54–61] Even some patients with pacemakers have died, probably because the atrium is so scarred that its stimulation is impossible.

If the patient has dilated cardiomyopathy, standard ACE-I treatment along with the other strategies defined earlier are appropriate. Ultimately, destination therapy and transplantation may be necessary.

LIMB-GIRDLE MUSCULAR DYSTROPHIES

Although the common presentation of shoulder and pelvic girdle weakness usually manifests in the teen years, several genetic types of limb-girdle muscular dystrophies (LGMD) exist. So far, 6 are autosomal dominant (LGMD 1A–1E) and 14 are autosomal recessive (LGMD 2A–2N), with a subset of 4 isoforms from sarcoglycan deficiency (LGMD 2D–2G).

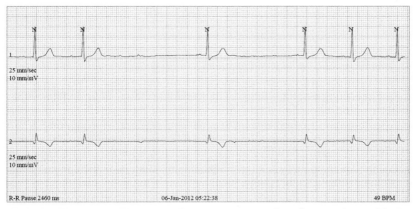

Fig. 6. Lack of P-wave capture on Holter monitor recording from patient with Emery-Dreifuss muscular dystrophy and cardiomyopathy. Pacemaker was placed.

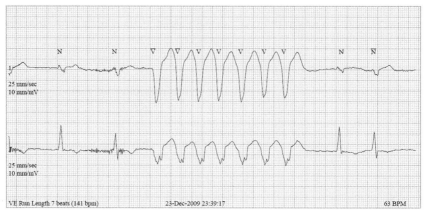

Fig. 7. Ventricular tachycardia in a patient with Emery-Dreifuss muscular dystrophy. n, normal beat; v, ventricular ectopic beat.

Cardiac Manifestations

Cardiomyopathy is more often seen in some of the sarcoglycan deficiencies and in LGMD 2I (defects in fukutin-related protein gene).[62–67] Cardiomyopathy is rare in the other types. Progressive conduction abnormalities are seen in LGMD 1B (Lamin A/C).

Treatment

Standard cardiomyopathy treatment is used. Destination therapy and transplantation may be necessary. Patients with heart block require pacemaker treatment.

FASCIOSCAPULAR MUSCULAR DYSTROPHY

Fascioscapular muscular dystrophy (FSHD) is one of the most common forms of muscular dystrophy. It is an autosomal dominant disorder mapping to chromosome 4q35 with a deletion in the D4Z4 repeat.[68] Patients have symmetric face, scapular stabilizer, and lower extremity muscular weakness of both the hip girdle and distal muscles.

Cardiac Involvement

Atrial and ventricular conduction defects can be seen but are extremely rare in FSHD.[69]

REFERENCES

1. Allen HD, Mendell JR, Hoffman TM. The Heart in muscular dystrophies. In: Allen HD, Driscoll DJ, Shaddy RE, et al, editors. Moss and Adams' heart disease in infants, children, and adolescents: including the fetus and young adult. 7th edition. Philadelphia: Wolters Kluwer/Lippincott Williams and Wilkins; 2008.
2. Allen HD, Flanigan KM, Mendell JR, et al. The Heart in muscular dystrophies. In: Allen HD, Driscoll DJ, Shaddy RE, et al, editors. Moss and Adams' heart disease in infants, children, and adolescents: including the fetus and young adult. 8th edition. Philadelphia: Wolters Kluwer/Lippincott Williams and Wilkins, in press.
3. Frankel KA, Rosser RJ. The pathology of the heart in progressive muscular dystrophy: epimyocardial fibrosis. Hum Pathol 1976;7:375–86.

4. Moriuchi T, Kagawa N, Mukoyama M, et al. Autopsy analyses of the muscular dystrophies. Tokushima J Exp Med 1993;40:83–93.
5. James TN. Observations of the cardiovascular involvement, including the cardiac conduction system, in progressive muscular dystrophy. Am Heart J 1962;63:48–56.
6. Hor KN, Wanasapura J, Markham LW, et al. Circumferential strain analysis identifies strata of cardiomyopathy in Duchenne muscular dystrophy. a cardiac magnetic resonance tagging study. J Am Coll Cardiol 2009;53:1204–10.
7. Puchalski MD, Williams RV, Askovich B, et al. Late gadolinium enhancement: precursor to cardiomyopathy in Duchenne muscular dystrophy? Int J Cardiovasc Imaging 2009;25:57–63.
8. Kaspar RW, Allen HD, Ray WC, et al. Analysis of dystrophin deletion mutations predicts age of cardiomyopathy onset in Becker muscular dystrophy. Circ Cardiovasc Genet 2009;2(6):544–51.
9. Shah AM, Jefferies JL, Rossano JW, et al. Electrocardiographic abnormalities and arrhythmias are strongly associated with the development of cardiomyopathy in muscular dystrophy. Heart Rhythm 2010;7:1484–8.
10. Perloff JK, Roberts WC, deLeon AC Jr. The distinctive electrocardiogram of Duchenne's progressive muscular dystrophy. An electrocardiographic-pathologic correlative study. Am J Med 1967;42:179–88.
11. Manning GW, Cropp GJ. The electrocardiogram in progressive muscular dystrophy. Br Heart J 1958;20:416.
12. Perloff JK. Cardiac rhythm and conduction in Duchenne's muscular dystrophy: a prospective study of 20 patients. J Am Coll Cardiol 1984;3:1263–8.
13. Bhattacharyya KB, Basu N, Ray TN, et al. Profile of electrocardiographic changes in Duchenne muscular dystrophy. J Indian Med Assoc 1997;95:40–2, 47.
14. Thrush PT, Allen HD, Viollet L, et al. Re-examination of the electrocardiogram in boys with Duchenne muscular dystrophy and correlation with its dilated cardiomyopathy. Am J Cardiol 2009;103:262–5.
15. Lanza GA, Dello Russo A, Giglio V, et al. Impairment of cardiac autonomic function in patients with Duchenne muscular dystrophy: relationship to myocardial and respiratory function. Am Heart J 2001;141:808–12.
16. Kirschmann C, Kececioglu D, Korinthenberg R, et al. Echocardiographic and electrocardiographic findings of cardiomyopathy in Duchenne and Becker-Kiener muscular dystrophies. Pediatr Cardiol 2005;26:66–72.
17. Vita G, DiLeo R, DeGregorio C, et al. Cardiovascular autonomic control in Becker muscular dystrophy. J Neurol Sci 2001;186:45–9.
18. Akita H, Matsuoka S, Kuroda Y. Predictive electrocardiographic score for evaluating prognosis in patients with Duchenne's muscular dystrophy. Tokushima J Exp Med 1993;40:55–60.
19. Chenard AA, Becane HM, Tertrain F, et al. Ventricular arrhythmia in Duchenne muscular dystrophy: prevalence, significance and prognosis. Neuromuscul Disord 1993;3:201–6.
20. Corrado G, Lissoni A, Beretta S, et al. Prognostic value of electrocardiograms, ventricular late potentials, ventricular arrhythmias, and left ventricular systolic dysfunction in patients with Duchenne muscular dystrophy. Am J Cardiol 2002;89:838–41.
21. Goldberg SJ, Feldman L, Reinecke C, et al. Echocardiographic determination of contraction and relaxation measurements of the left ventricular wall in normal subjects and patients with muscular dystrophy. Circulation 1980;62:1061–9.
22. Hunsaker RH, Fulkerson PK, Barry FJ, et al. Cardiac function in Duchenne's muscular dystrophy. Results of a 10-year follow-up study and noninvasive tests. Am J Med 1982;73:235–8.

23. Goldberg SJ, Stern LZ, Feldman L, et al. Serial two-dimensional echocardiography in Duchenne muscular dystrophy. Neurology 1982;32:1101–5.
24. Goldberg SJ, Stern LZ, Feldman L, et al. Serial left ventricular wall measurements in Duchenne's muscular dystrophy. J Am Coll Cardiol 1983;2:136–42.
25. Taneanaka A, Yokota M, Iwase M, et al. Discrepancy between systolic and diastolic dysfunction of the left ventricle in patients with Duchenne muscular dystrophy. Eur Heart J 1993;14:669–76.
26. Sasaki K, Sakata K, Kachi E, et al. Sequential changes in cardiac structure and function in patients with Duchenne type muscular dystrophy: a two-dimensional echocardiographic study. Am Heart J 1998;135:937–44.
27. Mori K, Edagawa T, Inoue M, et al. Peak negative myocardial velocity gradient and wall-thickening velocity during early diastole are noninvasive parameters of left ventricular diastolic function in patients with Duchenne's progressive muscular dystrophy. J Am Soc Echocardiogr 2004;17:322–9.
28. Mori K, Hayabuchi Y, Inoue M, et al. Myocardial strain imaging for early detection of cardiac involvement in patients with Duchenne's progressive muscular dystrophy. Echocardiography 2007;6:598–608.
29. Bosser G, Lucron H, Lethor JP, et al. Evidence of early impairments in both right and left ventricular inotropic reserves in children with Duchenne's muscular dystrophy. Am J Cardiol 2004;93:724–7.
30. Tani LY, Minich LL, Williams RV, et al. Ventricular remodeling in children with left ventricular dysfunction secondary to various cardiomyopathies. Am J Cardiol 2005;96:1157–61.
31. Yanagisawa A, Yokota N, Miyagawa M, et al. Plasma levels of atrial natriuretic peptide in patients with Duchenne's progressive muscular dystrophy. Am Heart J 1990;120:1154–8.
32. Mori K, Manabe T, Nii M, et al. Plasma levels of natriuretic peptide and echocardiographic parameters in patients with Duchenne's progressive muscular dystrophy. Pediatr Cardiol 2002;23:160–6.
33. Duboc D, Meune C, Lerebours G, et al. Effect of perindopril on the onset and progression of left ventricular dysfunction in Duchenne muscular dystrophy. J Am Coll Cardiol 2005;45:855–7.
34. Jefferies JL, Eidem BW, Belmont JW, et al. Genetic predictors and remodeling of dilated cardiomyopathy in muscular dystrophy. Circulation 2005;112:2799–804.
35. Naruse H, Miyagi J, Arii T, et al. The relationship between clinical stage, prognosis and myocardial damage in patients with Duchenne-type muscular dystrophy: five-year follow-up study. Ann Nucl Med 2004;18:203–8.
36. Stöllberger C, Finsterer J. Can perindopril delay the onset of heart failure in Duchenne muscular dystrophy? J Am Coll Cardiol 2005;46:1781.
37. Viollet L, Thrush PT, Flanigan KM, et al. Effects of angiotensin-converting enzyme inhibitors and/or β-blockers on the cardiomyopathy in Duchenne muscular dystrophy. Am J Cardiol 2012;110(1):98–102.
38. Duboc D, Meune C, Pierre B, et al. Perindopril preventive treatment on mortality in Duchenne muscular dystrophy: 10 years' follow-up. Am Heart J 2007;154: 596–602.
39. Rafael-Fortney JA, Chimanji NS, Schill KE, et al. Early treatment with lisinopril and spironolactone preserves cardiac and skeletal muscle in Duchenne muscular dystrophy mice. Circulation 2011;124:582–8.
40. Cripe LH, Barber BJ, Spicer RL, et al. Outpatient continuous inotrope infusion as an adjunct to heart failure therapy in Duchenne muscular dystrophy. Neuromuscul Disord 2006;16:745–8.

41. Buyse GM, Goemans N, van den Hauwe M, et al. Idebenone as a novel, thera-peutic approach for Duchenne muscular dystrophy: results from a 12 month, double-blind, randomized placebo-controlled trial. Neuromuscul Disord 2011; 21:396–405.

42. Breucking E, Reimnitz P, Schara U, et al. Anesthetic complications. The incidence of severe anesthetic complications in patients and families with progressive muscular dystrophy of the Duchenne and Becker types. Anaesthesist 2000;49: 187–95 [in German].

43. American Academy of Pediatrics Section on Cardiology and Cardiac Surgery. Cardiovascular health supervision for individuals affected by Duchenne or Beck-er muscular dystrophy. Pediatrics 2005;116:1569–73.

44. Sabovic M, Medica I, Logar N, et al. Relation of CTG expansion and clinical vari-ables to electrocardiogram conduction abnormalities and sudden death in patients with myotonic dystrophy. Neuromuscul Disord 2003;13:822–6.

45. Schara U, Schosser BG. Myotonic dystrophies type 1 & 2: a summary on current aspects. Semin Pediatr Neurol 2006;13:71–9.

46. Machuca-Tzili L, Brook D, Hilton-Jones D. Clinical and molecular aspects of the myotonic dystrophies: a review. Muscle Nerve 2005;32:1–18.

47. Steinert H. Uber das klinische und anatomische bild des muskelschwundes der myotoniker. Deutsche Ztschr Nervenh 1909;37:38–104 [in German].

48. Perloff JK, Stevenson WG, Roberts NK, et al. Cardiac involvement in myotonic muscular dystrophy (Steinert's disease): a prospective study of 25 patients. Am J Cardiol 1984;54:1074–81.

49. Finsterer J, Stöllberger C, Blazek G, et al. Cardiac involvement in myotonic dystrophy, Becker muscular dystrophy and mitochondrial myopathy: a five-year follow-up. Can J Cardiol 2001;17:1061–9.

50. Badano L, Autore C, Fragola PV, et al. Left ventricular myocardial function in myotonic dystrophy. Am J Cardiol 1993;71:987–91.

51. Vignaux O, Lazarus A, Varin J, et al. Right ventricular MR abnormalities in myotonic dystrophy and relationship with intracardiac electrophysiologic test findings: initial results. Radiology 2002;224:231–5.

52. Colleran JA, Hawley RJ, Pinnow EE, et al. Value of the electrocardiogram in determining cardiac events and mortality in myotonic dystrophy. Am J Cardiol 1997;80:1494–7.

53. Emery AE, Dreifuss FE. Unusual type of benign X-linked muscular dystrophy. J Neurol Neurosurg Psychiatry 1966;29:338–42.

54. Buckley AE, Dean J, Mahy IR. Cardiac involvement in Emery Dreifuss muscular dystrophy: a case series. Heart 1999;82:105–8.

55. Boriani G, Gallina M, Merlini L, et al. Clinical relevance of atrial fibrillation/flutter, stroke, pacemaker implant, and heart failure in Emery-Dreifuss muscular dystrophy: a long-term longitudinal study. Stroke 2003;34:901–8.

56. Becane HM, Bonne G, Varnous S, et al. High incidence of sudden death with conduction system and myocardial disease due to lamins A and C gene muta-tion. Pacing Clin Electrophysiol 2000;23:1661–6.

57. Bonne G, Mercuri E, Muchir A, et al. Clinical and molecular genetic spectrum of autosomal dominant Emery-Dreifuss muscular dystrophy due to mutations of the lamin A/C gene. Ann Neurol 2000;48:170–80.

58. Jakobs PM, Hanson EL, Crispell KA, et al. Novel lamin A/C mutations in two fami-lies with dilated cardiomyopathy and conduction system disease. J Card Fail 2001;7:249–56.

59. Sanna T, Dello Russo A, Toniolo D, et al. Cardiac features of Emery-Dreifuss muscular dystrophy caused by lamin A/C gene mutations. Eur Heart J 2003;24:2227–36.

60. Bialer MG, McDaniel NL, Kelly TE. Progression of cardiac disease in Emery-Dreifuss muscular dystrophy. Clin Cardiol 1991;14:411–6.

61. Yoshioka M, Saida K, Itagaki Y, et al. Follow up study of cardiac involvement in Emery-Dreifuss muscular dystrophy. Arch Dis Child 1989;64:713–5.

62. Beckmann JS, Bushby K. Advances in the molecular genetics of the limb-girdle type of autosomal recessive progressive muscular dystrophy. Curr Opin Neurol 1996;9:389–93.

63. Melacini P, Fanin M, Duggan DJ, et al. Heart involvement in muscular dystrophies due to sarcoglycan gene mutations. Muscle Nerve 1999;22:473–9.

64. Duggan DJ, Gorospe JR, Fanin M, et al. Mutations in the sarcoglycan genes in patients with myopathy. N Engl J Med 1997;336:618–24.

65. Wahbi K, Meune C, Hamouda el H, et al. Cardiac assessment of limb-girdle muscular dystrophy 2I patients: an echography, Holter ECG and magnetic resonance imaging study. Neuromuscul Disord 2008;18(8):650–5.

66. D'Amico A, Petrini S, Parisi F, et al. Heart transplantation in a child with LGMD2I presenting as isolated dilated cardiomyopathy. Neuromuscul Disord 2008;18(2): 153–5.

67. van der Kooi AJ, de Voogt WG, Barth PG, et al. The heart in limb girdle muscular dystrophy. Heart 1998;79:73–7.

68. Lemmers RJ, van der Vliet PJ, Klooster R, et al. A unifying genetic model for facioscapulohumeral muscular dystrophy. Science 2010;329(5999):1650–3.

69. Laforet P, de Toma C, Eymard B, et al. Cardiac involvement in genetically confirmed facioscapulohumeral muscular dystrophy. Neurology 1998;51:1454–6.

Treatment of Spine Deformity in Neuromuscular Diseases

Sukanta Maitra, MD[a], Rolando F. Roberto, MD[b],*,
Craig M. McDonald, MD[c], Munish C. Gupta, MD[b]

KEYWORDS

- Spinal deformity • Neuromuscular disease • Duchenne muscular dystrophy
- Spinal muscular atrophy • Surgical management

KEY POINTS

- Spinal deformity adversely affects the quality of life of patients with progressive hereditary neuromuscular diseases (NMDs).
- While the impact of spinal arthrodesis on pulmonary function remains controversial (the disease pathogenesis continues to affect chest wall muscles and diaphragm), there can be no doubt that failure to aggressively treat spinal deformity in progressive NMD can have profound negative consequences on sitting balance, pelvic obliquity, ability to sit comfortably in a wheelchair, cosmesis, and quality of life.
- There are emerging data that improvements in disease management in Duchenne muscular dystrophy (DMD) including treatment with corticosteroids, surgical management of spine deformity, noninvasive ventilation, and more effective treatment of cardiomyopathy have led to improved function and survival in DMD and a changing natural history of disease.
- Spinal arthrodesis with internal instrumentation is the only effective treatment, but optimally is deferred to the second decade so that anterior approaches are avoided. Spinal orthotics may be used in younger patients to provide postural support and more balanced sitting, but spinal orthotics generally do not affect the natural history of spinal deformity in NMD conditions.
- Surgical management of the spinal deformity often requires a multidisciplinary approach beginning in the preoperative surgical planning period owing to concomitant restrictive lung disease and cardiomyopathy in selected NMD conditions.

[a] Department of Orthopaedic Surgery, University of California Davis Med Center, 4860 Y Street, Suite 3800, Sacramento, CA 95817, USA; [b] Adult and Pediatric Spine Surgery, Department of Orthopaedic Surgery, University of California Davis, 4860 Y Street, Suite 3800, Sacramento, CA 95817, USA; [c] Department of Physical Medicine and Rehabilitation, University of California Davis School of Medicine, 4860 Y Street, Suite 3850, Sacramento, CA 95817, USA
* Corresponding author.
E-mail address: Rolando.roberto@ucdmc.ucdavis.edu

Phys Med Rehabil Clin N Am 23 (2012) 869–883
http://dx.doi.org/10.1016/j.pmr.2012.08.009
1047-9651/12/$ – see front matter © 2012 Elsevier Inc. All rights reserved.

INTRODUCTION

The treatment of pediatric scoliosis and kyphosis falls under 3 categories: idiopathic, congenital, and neuromuscular. The focus of this article is on neuromuscular spine deformity occurring in children with neuromuscular diseases (NMDs). In this context, NMDs are specifically defined by defects in function of the anterior horn cell (motor neuron diseases), the peripheral nerve system (neuropathies), the neuromuscular junction (congenital myasthenia), or muscles (eg, muscular dystrophies). For the spine surgeon, disease processes such as those that involve the central nervous system, such as cerebral palsy or spina bifida, are often combined into the umbrella term of neuromuscular scoliosis. However, this review focuses on pediatric diseases of the lower motor neuron (ie, NMDs) that are associated with spinal deformity.

Severe spinal deformity in progressive NMD leads to multiple problems, including poor sitting balance, difficulty with upright seating and positioning, pain, difficulty in attendant care, and potential exacerbation of underlying restrictive respiratory compromise. Severe scoliosis and pelvic obliquity can in some instances completely preclude upright sitting in a wheelchair. Aggressive management of spinal deformity with bracing and spinal instrumentation have been based on the assumption that progressive spinal deformity leads to poor sitting balance, pelvic obliquity, and greater likelihood of pressure sores, functional impairment, and poor cosmesis, as well as reduced quality of life.[1] While the impact of spinal arthrodesis on pulmonary function remains controversial (the disease pathogenesis continues to affect chest wall muscles and diaphragm), there can be no doubt that failure to aggressively treat spinal deformity in progressive NMD can have profound negative consequences on sitting balance, pelvic obliquity, ability to sit comfortably in a wheelchair, cosmesis, and quality of life (**Fig. 1**A). In addition, there are emerging data that improvements in disease management in Duchenne muscular dystrophy (DMD) including treatment with corticosteroids, surgical management of spine deformity, noninvasive ventilation, and more effective treatment of cardiomyopathy have led to improved function and survival in DMD and a changing disease natural history.[2–5]

PREVALENCE AND NATURAL HISTORY OF SPINAL DEFORMITY IN NMDS

Spinal deformity is a well-documented sequela of childhood-onset NMD and in some adults with NMD. The reported ultimate prevalence of scoliosis in DMD previously varied from 33% to 100% in the literature.[6–15] McDonald and colleagues[16] showed that 50% of males with DMD acquire scoliosis between 12 and 15 years of age, corresponding to the adolescent growth spurt. This study found that 10% of older DMD subjects showed no clinical scoliosis. This finding is consistent with that of Oda and colleagues[10] of a 15% prevalence of DMD patients with mild nonprogressive curves (usually 10°–30°). The rate of progression of the primary or single untreated curve has been reported to range from 11° to 42° per year, depending on the age span studied. Oda and colleagues[10] have shown that curve severity in the sagittal plane was a predictor of curve progression as well as pulmonary function changes over time. Most patients who developed progressive scoliosis showed less than 2000 mL peak obtained forced vital capacity (FVC). More recently, the incidence of scoliosis in DMD has been shown to be significantly reduced in those patients treated with glucocorticoids.[17–20]

Scoliosis has been estimated to occur in 78% to nearly 100% of patients with spinal muscular atrophy (SMA) type II.[21,22] Severity of weakness and age (skeletal maturity) have been described as critical factors influencing the risk for SMA patients of developing spinal deformity.[1] Scoliosis almost always begins in the first decade of life as

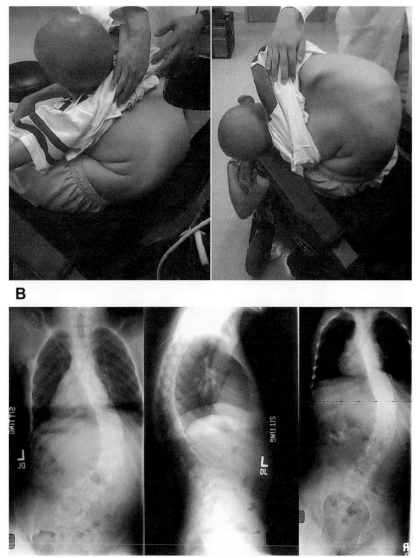

Fig. 1. (*A*) A 21-year-old man with Duchenne muscular dystrophy, glucocorticoid naïve for his entire life, on no medications, currently on no nocturnal or daytime noninvasive ventilation, and presenting for an initial evaluation in the Neuromuscular Disease Clinic at University of California Davis Medical Center in Sacramento, California. He has been cared for by an unidentified clinic outside the region in Southern California. The patient has severe spinal deformity and pelvic obliquity, and he is unable to sit comfortably in a manual wheelchair. Pulmonary function tests show that he has a percent predicted forced vital capacity of 18%, making spinal arthrodesis very high risk. (*B*) Preoperative radiographs of a young woman with diagnosis of spinal muscular atrophy (SMA). Sitting anteroposterior (AP) (*left*), sitting lateral (*middle*), and traction films (*right*). AP and lateral films provide insight into the plane of deformity (sagittal, coronal, or both) while traction films provide insight into flexibility of the curve. (*C*) Postoperative images of an SMA patient, with posterior segmental instrumentation illustrating proximal hook fixation with distal pedicle screw and iliac bolt fixation. Note the use of sublaminar wires placed along the rod in the concavity of the curve to assist in translation of the spine to improve coronal plane deformity. (Image *A Courtesy of* Craig McDonald, MD, UC Davis Medical Center.)

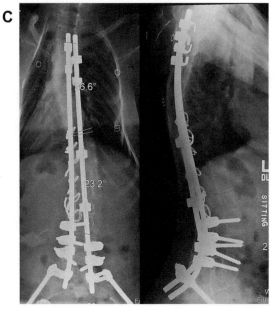

Fig. 1. (*continued*)

a result of sever truncal weakness. The curves are collapsing in nature, and may be thoracolumbar, thoracic, lumbar, double curves involving the thoracolumbar and thoracic regions, or double curves involving the thoracic and thoracolumbar regions.[1] In SMA, the average deformity is 90°, with a reported range from 20° to 164°. Severe kyphosis may be a common associated deformity, and almost all persons with severe scoliosis have significant pelvic obliquity. By contrast, patients with SMA type III who are still ambulating show a lower incidence of scoliosis, reported to be 8% to 63%.

In addition, spinal deformity has been shown by the authors' group to be common in severe childhood autosomal recessive limb-girdle muscular dystrophy (LGMD),[23] congenital muscular dystrophy,[1] and congenital myotonic muscular dystrophy.[24] Adults with facioscapulohumeral muscular dystrophy (FSHD) may develop collapsing hyperlordosis.[1] In 2 previous studies of the natural history of scoliosis in Friedreich ataxia, the prevalence of scoliosis approached 100%.[25,26]

CLINICAL MANAGEMENT OF NEUROMUSCULAR SCOLIOSIS

The early childhood period (age <8 years) is best managed with upright seating support allowing semirecumbent posture with lateral uprights to allow control of coronal plane collapse, and a wheelchair cushion providing weight transfer to the greatest surface area of the thigh. Early in the disease course of patients with scoliosis related to hypotonia, spinal curvatures are flexible and will completely correct with supine positioning. By contrast, upright radiographs (seated) will demonstrate global spinal collapse in the coronal plane and either kyphotic or lordotic collapse on the sagittal plane (lateral radiograph), which may depend on disease process or stage of disease. For children with spontaneous curve correction on supine radiographs, further observation and seating-support management is desirable. Young children with hypotonia and postural spine deformity may benefit from provision of a soft spinal orthosis to help with sitting balance.

For DMD patients the authors often obtain anteroposterior (AP) and lateral scoliosis films every 6 months between the ages of 11 and 16 for DMD, or earlier if they progress to full-time reliance on the wheelchair at a younger age. Curve progression can be unpredictable in this age group, and appropriate clinical surveillance is critical. It is not uncommon in this patient population to obtain regular pulmonary function tests (particularly for DMD) at least once if not twice a year during this critical age range to establish the peak FVC. Oda and colleagues[10] described an association between increased peak FVC and decreased curve progression in DMD patients. McDonald and colleagues[16] described DMD patients with peak FVC greater than 2.5 L/min to have milder disease progression than those with peak FVC less than 1.7 L/min. Therefore, use of peak FVC may act as a prognostic indicator for severity of spinal deformity in DMD. Radiographic surveillance begins earlier in patients with SMA II, owing to the earlier onset of spine deformity.

Spinal Bracing for Management of Spine Deformity in NMD

The use of orthosis in the management of spinal deformity has been studied extensively.[6,27,28] The use of orthotics is generally poorly tolerated by the neuromuscular patient population, and may create a situation whereby the FVC can be lowered with these devices unless care is taken to provide an anterior soft opening to accommodate chest-wall expansion and abdominal protuberance caused by predominant diaphragm breathing patterns. Bracing has been proved to be ineffective, with no clear evidence in the literature that orthotics prevent progression of spinal deformity in the NMD patient population. If bracing is prescribed in a patient with NMD, the indication is usually the need for a soft thoraco-lumbo-sacral orthosis to help with sitting balance. In SMA type II, prophylactic bracing has been used by many clinicians to delay the development of spinal deformity to the second decade and/or decrease the severity of deformity so that the child can grow as much as possible before spinal fusion. Even in patients with adolescent idiopathic scoliosis, bracing continues to be controversial. For example, Negrini and colleagues,[28] in a Cochrane review of bracing in adolescent idiopathic scoliosis, were unable to draw definitive conclusions regarding bracing based on the lack of data from randomized control studies that used the Scoliosis Research Society (SRS) guidelines for study. In other words, a meta-analysis could not be performed for lack of appropriate level of evidence in the literature. The authors' clinical experience shows that bracing can improve younger NMD patient's sitting posture once curve progression has occurred, while being are aware that it may not obviate surgical intervention.

In a majority of neuromuscular patients with scoliosis, the lumbar and thoracolumbar spine serves as the apex or focus of spinal deformity, with a resultant truncal decompensation. Impaired sitting balance also occurs related to pelvic obliquity, which when present is frequently rigid and not well compensated for by alterations in seating (custom or compensated seat cushioning). In these children and adolescents, excessive tilt is noted by parents and caregivers. More commonly the coronal plane deformity is accompanied by a kyphotic sagittal plane alignment that also interferes with upright sitting posture. It is relatively common for patients and caregivers to relate back-pain complaints as scoliosis worsens. Previous guidelines in neuromuscular patients recommended surgical treatment for scoliosis once angular deformity exceeded 25°, citing an optimal match between Cobb angle as predictive of relentless progression with favorable pulmonary volumes.[29]

Because of recent advances in pediatric critical care management and postoperative respiratory therapy support, surgical treatment of spine deformity in DMD can be deferred until Cobb angle measurements approach 45° to 50° and may be safely tolerated in patients with FVC measurements even below 30% to 40% predicted.[30] In the authors' recently published series on DMD,[31] operative intervention was performed on patients of average age approximately 12 years with average curve size of 47°. The greatest curve seen in this series, however, measured more than 100°, reflecting the potential for curves to behave rather poorly and contribute to patient morbidity and discomfort. In this patient cohort, which spanned approximately 2 decades, long-term surgical correction averaged 50% using methods that have evolved more recently, owing to the advances in spinal implant technology. In our experience, more modern techniques of screw fixation and anchorage with iliac bolts to the pelvis demonstrate greater correction (>66%) and near complete correction of pelvic obliquity.

PERIOPERATIVE PLANNING
Preoperative Workup

For any surgical procedure, an appropriate history and physical examination must be obtained, as well as an understanding of the patient's or the family's expectations from the surgery (ie, improved sitting posture vs cosmetic correction). In addition, the assistance of a pediatrician to ensure the patient is medically optimized for surgery is very helpful. For instance, assessing the appropriate nutritional status of the patient (eg, obtaining complete metabolic panel, and prealbumin, and albumin levels) is critical for possible wound-healing complications, but may require the use of gastrostomy-tube placement preoperatively in severely nutritionally deficient patients. In addition, cardiomyopathy is progressive in the cohort of patients with DMD, although rarely is ejection fraction impaired to the level precluding surgical management of scoliosis. A prolonged impressive tachycardia is commonly seen in the DMD patient preoperatively because of the effects of dystrophin on the autonomic nervous system. Close cardiac monitoring and pulmonary interventions during the immediate postoperative period (48–72 hours) require critical care support. Preoperative cardiology consultation is helpful to assess ejection fraction and to preclude the more uncommon aberrant pathways and conduction anomalies that may be seen with involvement of Purkinje fibers. Echocardiograms and electrocardiograms are routinely obtained in these patients.

In their institutional experience with appropriate patient selection and postoperative pediatric critical care management aided by excellent anesthetic care, the authors have noted that the average length of time intubated postoperatively is less than a day and the average stay in the intensive care unit is between 2 and 3 days. All patients and families are counseled about the potential need for prolonged mechanical ventilation, the risk for postoperative pneumonias, and the remote possibility that tracheostomy may be required should weaning from mechanical ventilation be prolonged in time course.

Preoperative Radiographic Workup

AP and lateral scoliosis films are obtained along with traction and bending films, which assist in determining flexibility of the curve and the appropriate levels for instrumentation (see **Fig. 1**B; **Figs. 2**A, B and **3**A). A majority of neuromuscular scoliosis can be treated with posterior spinal instrumentation and fusion from T3 to the pelvis. However, in the case of an extremely rigid curve, the need for an anterior/posterior procedure is required to achieve adequate correction. Preoperative computed tomography scans may be used specifically to ascertain the bony anatomy for placement of spinal instrumentation. The use of preoperative magnetic resonance imaging is reserved for those cases whereby spinal cord abnormalities are suspected.

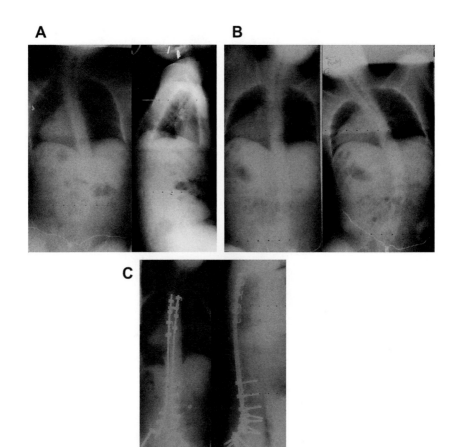

Fig. 2. (A) Preoperative images of young man with Duchenne muscular dystrophy (DMD). Note the coronal and sagittal plane deformities on the AP and lateral view. (B) Preoperative bending films illustrate the flexibility of curve and often guide treatment: for example, posterior-only approach for flexible curves versus combination anterior/posterior approach for more rigid curves. (C) Postoperative films of a DMD patient with improvement in sagittal and coronal plane. The patient underwent a posterior-only approach secondary to the flexibility of the curve noted in the preoperative bending films.

Intraoperative

The authors recommend preoperative antibiotics at least 1 hour before surgery, to be continued for 48 hours postoperatively. The antibiotics used depend on the local sensitivities of *Staphylococcus* and *Streptococcus* species. The authors routinely use cephalosporins such as cefazolin for empiric coverage against these species, in addition to using vancomycin for additional prophylaxis against methicillin-resistant *Staphylococcus aureus*. Intraoperative cord monitoring with somatosensory evoked potentials is used as well as Cell Saver. Operative intervention for the treatment of the scoliotic curves generally requires treatment with instrumentation and fusion of the majority of the spine, and requires anchorage to the pelvis. In DMD, given the large intervention and the presence of dystrophin in the capillaries, blood loss is significant and usually amounts to half to one full circulating blood volume

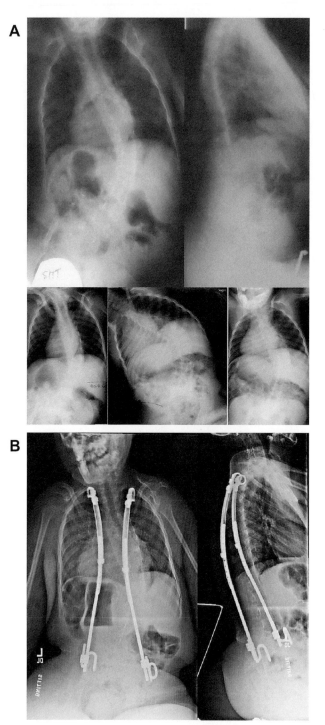

Fig. 3. (*A*) Preoperative films including AP/lateral, bending films, and traction film undergoing growing-rod treatment. Based on the flexibility of the patient's curve and relatively young age, the use of a growing-rod construct was deemed best for this patient. (*B*) Postoperative films illustrating use of vertical expandable prosthetic titanium rib (VEPTR) as growing rods. Placement of dual growing rods occurs at the same levels as the definitive fusion. The goal is to maintain correction of the scoliosis while allowing the spine to continue to grow before definitive fusion surgery.

(2–5 L estimated blood loss). Most anesthesia protocols recommend use of antifibrinolytic drugs (transexemic acid or ε-aminocaproic acid), a recommendation fully supported by the authors.

Postoperative

Patients are observed in the intensive care unit for at least 24 hours after surgery. The main concern is that of pulmonary toilet postoperatively. Adequate pain control in the postoperative period is managed with use of patient-controlled analgesia pumps or providing around-the-clock intravenous narcotics by nursing if necessary. If patients remain ventilated, respiratory therapy is initiated immediately postoperatively, including intrapulmonary percussive ventilation (IPV) or intermittent positive-pressure breathing (IPPB) to increase pulmonary toilet, improve mobilization of secretions, and prevent atelectasis. Patients may be extubated to noninvasive ventilation with bilevel positive airway pressure, and in addition they may use IPV, IPPB, or the cough assist machine. Physical therapists ensure patients are mobilized while in bed and out of bed, to improve pulmonary toilet and prevent further muscle wasting or contractures.

OPERATIVE TECHNIQUE

Historically, spinal stabilization occurred through Harrington rod constructs; however, the use of the distraction system provided only 2 points of fixation and required postoperative external immobilization for best results. Moreover, the Harrington rod system required extensive decortication and autogenous bone grafting, and more often than not was prone to curve progression and pseudoarthrosis.[32,33] By the mid-1970s Luque[34,35] began the process of segmental spinal instrumentation using sublaminar wires, and ultimately described improved correction rates and pseudarthrosis rates.[34,35] However, as one can imagine, the technique often did not address the issue of pelvic obliquity and instability through the lumbosacral region of this particular patient population. The next logical step was attributable to the work of Allen and Ferguson,[36] who pioneered the Galveston technique. This technique still used the segmental spinal instrumentation as described by Luque; however, for pelvic fixation the Luque rods were bent and passed intraosseously in the ileum, passing from the lower margin of the posterior superior iliac spine across the posterior column and into the transverse bar of the ilium.[36] The disadvantages of this technique involved the precision required to bend the rods appropriately, with imperfection leading to loss of correction and pseudarthrosis. The investigators reported an increase in operative time as well. More recent clinical data suggest that there is an associated loss of sagittal plane correction along with high incidence of proximal fixation pullout and distal migration of the rods, as described by Sink and colleagues.[37]

Even to this day there is debate in the literature regarding the use of instrumentation to the pelvis in neuromuscular patients.[38–40] The authors use spinopelvic fixation to anchor the long fusion and to provide correction to pelvic obliquity if it exists (see **Figs.** 1C and 2C). The latest evolution of the spinal instrumentation is the use of segmental fixation (pedicle screws, laminar hooks, and sublaminar wires) known as the Isola-Galveston technique. Yazici and colleagues,[41] in a retrospective review of 47 neuromuscular patients (the majority with cerebral palsy) with an average of 4-year follow-up, described 66% correction of scoliosis (70°–24°) and an 81% correction of pelvic obliquity (27°–5°) with an overall pseudarthrosis rate of 9%. These results were much improved when compared with a similar population using the Galveston technique.[42]

Refinements to the segmental instrumentation of neuromuscular patients included use of iliac bolts and/or screws using rod connectors as opposed to manipulating the rod itself to provide pelvic fixation.[43,44] For example, Peelle and colleagues[44] described, in a retrospective review of 40 total neuromuscular patients (20 patients for the Galveston and 20 for iliac and lumbosacral screw technique), an improvement in pelvic obliquity and in the radiographic finding of radiolucent halos surrounding the pelvic anchor. In other words, an equally rigid construct is created without the need for bending the rod in 3 dimensions or the need for replacing entire constructs if there is rod breakage.

Although the use of the anterior approach and release is generally advantageous for achieving significant levels of correction for rigid and significant curves, in the neuromuscular population with restrictive pulmonary disease, anterior procedures are generally avoided because of the inherent complications associated with procedures involving the diaphragm. Anterior releases performed in the first decade help prevent the crankshaft phenomenon or further rotatory deformity in the younger neuromuscular patients, but the procedure has inherent risks in NMD. The anterior approach and release is particularly risky near the upper thoracic region where involvement of the diaphragm in the procedure can lead to decreased FVC in the postoperative period, thus leading to increased atelectasis, poor pulmonary toilet, potential pneumonias, and prolonged mechanical ventilation. The anterior approach, therefore, is rarely used the NMD patient population.

The posterior approach requires adequate exposure of the posterior spine, which must occur with subperiosteal dissection of the spinous processes and lamina down to the facets. Placement of the proximal and distal fixation points or anchors follows with placement of screws, laminar hooks, and/or transverse process hooks proximally and pedicle screws distally, with the placement of iliac bolts. Once anchor points are inserted, the next step involves translating and rotating the spine to the sagittally contoured rods. Often the use of a cantilever technique (ie, fixing separate rods proximally and distally and bringing the free ends to the opposite ends) may assist in providing the majority of the correction necessary. Translation is aided by preinserting the sublaminar wires in the thoracic spine and tying them to the rod on the concavity of the curve (see **Fig. 1**C). The benefit of the segmental instrumentation technique is that adjustments such as distraction and compression can be made once the rods are in place to ensure maximal correction in the coronal plane as well as for pelvic obliquity. This maneuver is then followed by final tightening of instrumentation, decortication of the posterior elements using a high-speed burr, and placement of local autogenous graft and allograft chips.

Often patients with NMD require surgical intervention within the first decade of life, which may be difficult in terms of the maturity of the thorax as well as their ultimate sitting height. The creation of growing-rod systems has allowed for intervention without the need for fusion, thus allowing for correction of scoliosis while allowing for continued spinal growth. Moe and colleagues[45] were one of the first to describe the distraction of the growing spine using Harrington rods and external bracing without fusion in 20 patients between 1973 and 1981. As the technology of the distraction system evolved, including lower profile implants to bisegmental claws on both ends and using 2 rods versus 1, the application in a variety of early-onset scoliosis cases increased. In a multicenter study, Akbarnia and colleagues[46] described the use of a dual-rod technique for the treatment of 23 heterogeneous patients from 1993 to 2001 who had early-onset scoliosis (curve progression greater than 10° despite nonoperative management) with a mean age at time of surgery of 5.4 years. The investigators report maintenance of correction following initial surgery compared with final follow-up or after final fusion, as well as statistical significance in measurements of space available for lung in 14 patients with thoracic scoliosis from preoperative status to final follow-up.

For the growing-rod technique, similar principles to those described earlier are used with the correction of curves from the posterior approach, with the exception of using smaller incisions at the proximal and distal fixation points and placement of the rods subcutaneously. The proximal and distal points of fixation are exposed in subperiosteal fashion, and proximal fixation is usually through hooks (typically in the region of T3–T4 for neuromuscular patients), while distally either hooks or screws can be used for fixation. The levels both proximally and distally are the levels one would choose for final fixation (see **Fig. 3**B). Once proximal and distal fixation points are in place, rods are contoured, and using a cantilever and torsion maneuver the rods are connected to a growing connector over the thoracolumbar junction. Combination of distraction forces on the concavity and compression forces on the convexity of the curve are used to obtain a balanced spine. The rods and connectors are placed within the paravertebral musculature and closed. Rods are lengthened every 6 months on average.

COMPLICATIONS

Like any scoliosis surgery, infections, bleeding, injury to the spinal cord, and cardiac or respiratory events are all very much significant concerns in this patient population. Mohamad and colleagues,[47] in a retrospective review of 175 patients undergoing surgery for neuromuscular scoliosis, reported a 33% complication rate. Modi and colleagues,[48] in a retrospective review of 50 neuromuscular patients, described a 68% complication rate. In the study by Reames and colleagues[49] of the SRS database of 4657 neuromuscular scoliosis cases of 19,360 scoliosis surgeries, there was an 18% complication rate compared with 10% for congenital scoliosis and 6% for idiopathic scoliosis. In addition, when the data was stratified in this cohort to include primary versus revision surgery, there was no statistical difference in associated complications between primary or revision surgery in the neuromuscular group.

Given that the vast majority of these children have not been able to perform any weight-bearing exercise and a subset has been exposed to long-term corticosteroid administration, there is a potential for perioperative long bone fracture. The authors have uncommonly seen fractures of the hip and humerus associated with careful positioning of patients with upper extremity and lower extremity contractures, and suspect that occasionally patients may sustain fractures of the ribs with intraoperative positioning. As many patients with DMD are obese earlier in their disease course, wound infections may occur at a rate as high as 10%, which has been seen in other neuromuscular patient populations.[50]

Dysphagia and aspiration seem to be rare in DMD, but cachexia can be associated with early death. Weight loss in DMD can commonly be attributed to inadequate caloric intake caused by loss of ability to self-feed and/or fatigue. A recent clinical investigation evaluated whether scoliosis in DMD repair is associated with malnutrition.[51] A retrospective chart review was undertaken of patients with DMD, including those who underwent operative repair of scoliosis. The investigators identified 9 boys who lost greater than 5% of body weight within 12 months of surgery and 8 patients who gained weight after surgery. Eight patients of comparable age who had no surgery served as control subjects. All patients had no change in biceps strength after surgery, but those who lost weight were unable to self-feed. Weight loss after surgery was associated with loss of self-feeding. It was concluded that preoperative and postoperative management of patients with DMD should include feeding evaluation and determination of postural changes associated with the spine fusion.

Postoperative functional limitations can also be seen. As fixation of the entirety of the spine to the pelvis would preclude ambulation in the previously ambulatory patient, the authors do not recommend surgical intervention in this patient population until patients have become wheelchair sitters. Several investigators report a decline in some functional activities in persons with SMA after spinal arthrodesis/fusion including gross motor skills, transfer ability, self-feeding, hygiene, dressing, independent toileting, and ambulation.[52–54] These declines were usually seen in weaker patients, and similar reductions in function were predicted with continued curve progression. For example, the most common postoperative functional deficit seen in the Duchenne population treated surgically is greater postoperative difficulty in self-feeding than preoperatively.[51] The elongation of the torso with decreased flexibility exacerbates the effects of upper extremity weakness, and additional adaptations are required to allow patients to effectively perform hand-to-mouth activities. Often a tray is required to rest the elbows postoperatively for these patients.

SUMMARY

Spinal deformity may adversely affect the quality of life in several progressive NMDs. Effective management requires an understanding of the age of onset and natural history of spinal deformity in specific neuromuscular diseases. Spinal arthrodesis with internal instrumentation is the only effective treatment, but optimally is deferred to the second decade so that anterior approaches are avoided. Spinal orthotics may be used in younger patients to provide postural support and more balanced sitting, but spinal orthotics generally do not affect the natural history of spinal deformity in NMD conditions. Growing-rod systems are options in younger patients to avoid early fusions that would severely compromise sitting height. Surgical management of the spinal deformity often requires a multidisciplinary approach beginning in the preoperative surgical planning period, owing to concomitant restrictive lung disease and cardiomyopathy in selected NMD conditions. The need for thorough and thoughtful discussions must occur with the family and other caregivers before any scheduled surgery. The decision to proceed with spinal instrumentation may alter functional abilities in marginally ambulatory FSHD patients or SMA III patients with proximal weakness with hyperlordosis; this also holds true for more severely affected NMD patients, such as those with SMA II, who may benefit functionally from greater flexibility of the spine for positioning of weak extremities. The impact of spinal instrumentation on life expectancy for more severe NMD conditions such as DMD, autosomal recessive LGMD, congenital muscular dystrophy, and SMA type II is a matter of some controversy and warrants further study. The care and treatment of persons with NMD and spinal deformity can be challenging, but with a multidisciplinary team, proper planning, and support, the patients will likely experience rewarding outcomes and improved quality of life.

REFERENCES

1. Hart DA, McDonald CM. Spinal deformity in progressive neuromuscular disease: natural history and management. Phys Med Rehabil Clin N Am 1999;9(1):213–32, viii.
2. Brooke MH, Fenichel GM, Griggs RC, et al. Clinical investigation in Duchenne dystrophy: 2. Determination of the "power" of therapeutic trials based on the natural history. Muscle Nerve 1983;6(2):91–103.

3. Eagle M, Baudouin SV, Chandler C, et al. Survival in Duchenne muscular dystrophy: improvements in life expectancy since 1967 and the impact of home nocturnal ventilation. Neuromuscul Disord 2002;12(10):926–9.

4. Bushby K, Finkel R, Birnkrant DJ, et al. Diagnosis and management of Duchenne muscular dystrophy, part 1: diagnosis, and pharmacological and psychosocial management. Lancet Neurol 2010;9(1):77–93.

5. Bushby K, Finkel R, Birnkrant DJ, et al. Diagnosis and management of Duchenne muscular dystrophy, part 2: implementation of multidisciplinary care. Lancet Neurol 2010;9(2):177–89.

6. Cambridge W, Drennan JC. Scoliosis associated with Duchenne muscular dystrophy. J Pediatr Orthop 1987;7(4):436–40.

7. Galasko CS. Incidence of orthopedic problems in children with muscle disease. Isr J Med Sci 1977;13(2):165–76.

8. Hsu JD. The natural history of spine curvature progression in the nonambulatory Duchenne muscular dystrophy patient. Spine (Phila Pa 1976) 1983;8(7):771–5.

9. Lord J, Behrman B, Varzos N, et al. Scoliosis associated with Duchenne muscular dystrophy. Arch Phys Med Rehabil 1990;71(1):13–7.

10. Oda T, Shimizu N, Yonenobu K, et al. Longitudinal study of spinal deformity in Duchenne muscular dystrophy. J Pediatr Orthop 1993;13(4):478–88.

11. Pecak F, Trontelj JV, Dimitrijevic MR. Scoliosis in neuromuscular disorders. Int Orthop 1980;3(4):323–8.

12. Robin GC, Brief LP. Scoliosis in childhood muscular dystrophy. J Bone Joint Surg Am 1971;53(3):466–76.

13. Sakai DN, Hsu JD, Bonnett CA, et al. Stabilization of the collapsing spine in Duchenne muscular dystrophy. Clin Orthop Relat Res 1977 Oct;(128):256–60.

14. Smith AD, Koreska J, Moseley CF. Progression of scoliosis in Duchenne muscular dystrophy. J Bone Joint Surg Am 1989;71(7):1066–74.

15. Wilkins KE, Gibson DA. The patterns of spinal deformity in Duchenne muscular dystrophy. J Bone Joint Surg Am 1976;58(1):24–32.

16. McDonald CM, Abresch RT, Carter GT, et al. Profiles of neuromuscular diseases: Duchenne muscular dystrophy. Am J Phys Med Rehabil 1995;74(Suppl 5): S70–92.

17. Biggar WD, Harris VA, Eliasoph L, et al. Long-term benefits of deflazacort treatment for boys with Duchenne muscular dystrophy in their second decade. Neuromuscul Disord 2006;16(4):249–55.

18. Balaban B, Matthews DJ, Clayton GH, et al. Corticosteroid treatment and functional improvement in Duchenne muscular dystrophy: long-term effect. Am J Phys Med Rehabil 2005;84(11):843–50.

19. Biggar WD, Politano L, Harris VA, et al. Deflazacort in Duchenne muscular dystrophy: a comparison of two different protocols. Neuromuscul Disord 2004; 14(8–9):476–82.

20. Alman BA, Raza SN, Biggar WD. Steroid treatment and the development of scoliosis in males with Duchenne muscular dystrophy. J Bone Joint Surg Am 2004; 86-A(3):519–24.

21. Granata C, Merlini L, Magni E, et al. Spinal muscular atrophy: natural history and orthopaedic treatment of scoliosis. Spine (Phila Pa 1976) 1989;14(7):760–2.

22. Carter GT, Abresch RT, Fowler WM, et al. Profiles of neuro-muscular diseases: spinal muscular atrophy. Am J Phys Med Rehabil 1995;74(5 Suppl):S150–9.

23. McDonald CM, Johnson ER, Abresch RT, et al. Profiles of neuro-muscular diseases: limb girdle syndromes. Am J Phys Med Rehabil 1995;74(Suppl 5): S117–30.

24. Johnson ER, Abresch RT, Carter GT, et al. Profiles of neuromuscular diseases. Myotonic dystrophy. Am J Phys Med Rehabil 1995;74(Suppl 5): S104–16.
25. Cady RB, Bobechko WP. Incidence, natural history, and treatment of scoliosis in Friedreich's ataxia. J Pediatr Orthop 1984;4(6):673–6.
26. Labelle H, Tohmé S, Duhaime M, et al. Natural history of scoliosis in Friedreich's ataxia. J Bone Joint Surg Am 1986;68(4):564–72.
27. Daher YH, Lonstein JE, Winter RB, et al. Spinal surgery in spinal muscular atrophy. J Pediatr Orthop 1985;5(4):391–5.
28. Negrini S, Minozzi S, Bettany-Saltikov J, et al. Braces for idiopathic scoliosis in adolescents [review]. Cochrane Database Syst Rev 2010;(1):CD006850.
29. Kurz LT, Mubarak SJ, Schultz P, et al. Correlation of scoliosis and pulmonary function in Duchenne muscular dystrophy. J Pediatr Orthop 1983;3:347–53.
30. Takaso M, Nakazawa T, Imura T, et al. Surgical management of severe scoliosis with high risk pulmonary dysfunction in Duchenne muscular dystrophy: patient function, quality of life and satisfaction. Int Orthop 2010;34(5):695–702.
31. Roberto R, Fritz A, Hagar Y, et al. The natural history of cardiac and pulmonary function decline in patients with Duchenne muscular dystrophy. Spine (Phila Pa 1976) 2011;36(15):E1009–17.
32. Bonnett C, Brown JC, Perry J, et al. Evolution of treatment of paralytic scoliosis at Rancho Los Amigos Hospital. J Bone Joint Surg Am 1975;57(2):206–15.
33. Bonnett C, Brown JC, Grow T. Thoracolumbar scoliosis in cerebral palsy. Results of surgical treatment. J Bone Joint Surg Am 1976;58(3):328–36.
34. Luque ER. Segmental spinal instrumentation for correction of scoliosis. Clin Orthop Relat Res 1982 Mar;(163):192–8.
35. Luque ER. The anatomic basis and development of segmental spinal instrumentation. Spine (Phila Pa 1976) 1982;7(3):256–9.
36. Allen BL Jr, Ferguson RL. The Galveston technique for L rod instrumentation of the scoliotic spine. Spine (Phila Pa 1976) 1982;7(3):276–84.
37. Sink EL, Newton PO, Mubarak SJ, et al. Maintenance of sagittal plane alignment after surgical correction of spinal deformity in patients with cerebral palsy. Spine (Phila Pa 1976) 2003;28(13):1396–403.
38. Mubarak SJ, Morin WD, Leach J. Spinal fusion in Duchenne muscular dystrophy fixation and fusion to the sacropelvis. J Pediatr Orthop 1993;13(6):752–7.
39. Sengupta DK, Mehdian SH, McConnell JR, et al. Pelvic or lumbar fixation for the surgical management of scoliosis in Duchenne muscular dystrophy. Spine 2002; 27(18):2072–9.
40. Gaine WJ, Lim J, Stephenson W, et al. Progression of scoliosis after spinal fusion in Duchenne's muscular dystrophy. J Bone Joint Surg Br 2004;86(4):550–5.
41. Yazici M, Asher MA, Hardacker JW. The safety and efficacy of Isola-Galveston instrumentation and arthrodesis in the treatment of neuromuscular spinal deformities. J Bone Joint Surg Am 2000;82(4):524–43.
42. Gau YL, Lonstein JE, Winter RB, et al. Luque-Galveston procedure for correction and stabilization of neuromuscular scoliosis and pelvic obliquity: a review of 68 patients. J Spinal Disord 1991;4:399–410.
43. Phillips JH, Gutheil JP, Knapp DR Jr. Iliac screw fixation in neuromuscular scoliosis. Spine (Phila Pa 1976) 2007;32(14):1566–70.
44. Peelle MW, Lenke LG, Bridwell KH, et al. Comparison of pelvic fixation techniques in neuromuscular spinal deformity correction: Galveston rod versus iliac and lumbosacral screws. Spine (Phila Pa 1976) 2006;31(20):2392–8 [discussion: 2399].

45. Moe JH, Kharrat K, Winter RB, et al. Harrington instrumentation without fusion plus external orthotic support for the treatment of difficult curvature problems in young children. Clin Orthop Relat Res 1984 May;(185):35–45.
46. Akbarnia BA, Marks DS, Boachie-Adjei O, et al. Dual growing rod technique for the treatment of progressive early-onset scoliosis: a multicenter study. Spine 2005;30:S46–57.
47. Mohamad F, Parent S, Pawelek J, et al. Perioperative complications after surgical correction in neuromuscular scoliosis. J Pediatr Orthop 2007;27(4):392–7.
48. Modi HN, Suh SW, Yang JH, et al. Surgical complications in neuromuscular scoliosis operated with posterior- only approach using pedicle screw fixation. Scoliosis 2009;4:11.
49. Reames DL, Smith JS, Fu KM, et al, Scoliosis Research Society Morbidity and Mortality Committee. Complications in the surgical treatment of 19,360 cases of pediatric scoliosis: a review of the Scoliosis Research Society Morbidity and Mortality database. Spine (Phila Pa 1976) 2011;36(18):1484–91.
50. Perry JW, Montgomerie JZ, Swank S, et al. Wound infections following spinal fusion with posterior segmental spinal instrumentation. Clin Infect Dis 1997; 24(4):558–61.
51. Iannaccone ST, Owens H, Scott J, et al. Postoperative malnutrition in Duchenne muscular dystrophy. J Child Neurol 2003;18(1):17–20.
52. Brown JC, Zeller JL, Swank SM, et al. Surgical and functional results of spine fusion in spinal muscular atrophy. Spine 1989;14:763–70.
53. Furumasu J, Swank SM, Brown JC, et al. Functional activities in spinal muscular atrophy patients after spinal fusion. Spine (Phila Pa 1976) 1989;14(7):771–5.
54. Schwentker EP, Gibson DA. The orthopaedic aspects of spinal muscular atrophy. J Bone Joint Surg Am 1976;58(1):32–8.

Mobility-Assistive Technology in Progressive Neuromuscular Disease

Wendy Lin, MD[a], Aaron Pierce, MS, ATP[b],
Andrew J. Skalsky, MD[c,d],*, Craig M. McDonald, MD[e]

KEYWORDS

- Neuromuscular disease • Mobility • Environmental control • Seating • Positioning

KEY POINTS

- Children as young as 24 months can learn to safely operate a power wheelchair.
- Power-assist wheelchairs are useful for nonambulatory patients with neuromuscular disease (NMD) with mild upper limb weakness.
- The NMD multidisciplinary team needs to consider the specific neuromuscular disease and plan for appropriate progression affecting the need for modifiable mobility devices.
- Proper seating and positioning is critical to maximize function and the optimal use of mobility-assistive technologies.
- Electronic control systems are available to integrate with environmental control systems and computer access.

INTRODUCTION

Mobility-assistive technology is essential for maintaining the function of individuals with severe or progressive neuromuscular disease (NMD). The types of devices required change as the disease progresses. In the pediatric population, despite disease progression, there can still be developmental progress in a variety of cognitive and social domains. Without proper accommodations for goal-directed independent mobility whereby children can explore and affect their environment, there can be delays in cognitive and social development caused by mobility impairment.[1] These devices need to be able to accommodate and adapt to the individual's needs.

[a] Department of Pediatrics, University of California San Diego, San Diego, CA, USA; [b] Independent Consultant, 429 Durian Street, Vista, San Diego, CA 92083, USA; [c] Pediatric Rehabilitation Program, University of California San Diego School of Medicine, San Diego, CA, USA; [d] Pediatric Rehabilitation Medicine, Rady Children's Hospital, 3020 Children's Way, MC 5096, San Diego, CA 92123, USA; [e] Department of Physical Medicine and Rehabilitation, University of California Davis School of Medicine, 4860 "Y" Street, Sacramento, CA 95817, USA
* Corresponding author. Pediatric Rehabilitation Medicine, 3020 Children's Way MC 5096, San Diego, CA 92123.
E-mail address: askalsky@rchsd.org

Phys Med Rehabil Clin N Am 23 (2012) 885–894
http://dx.doi.org/10.1016/j.pmr.2012.08.007
1047-9651/12/$ – see front matter © 2012 Elsevier Inc. All rights reserved.
pmr.theclinics.com

As more specialized functions are required, the financial cost also increases. It is important for the clinician, therapist, family, and patient to be aware of what durable medical equipment coverage is available as well as the qualification for such equipment based on medical necessity and documentation requirements imposed by their specific funding source. Coverage, qualification based on medical necessity, and documentation requirements vary by payer source and region. It is also important to consider charitable resources that can provide assistance when needed.

Required considerations for the proper evaluation of mobility-assistive technology include a physical, visual, and cognitive assessment. The evaluation frequency needs to be completed based on the functional status of the patient and the rate and degree of disease progression. Physical, occupational, and speech therapists can be involved to provide insights regarding the interface between the patient and the device. These insights may influence the decision to choose a particular product rather than another. Overall, there needs to be a patient-centered team approach when addressing the needs of this patient population to determine what type of device is most appropriate.

MOBILITY-ASSISTIVE TECHNOLOGY IN THE PEDIATRIC NMD POPULATION

Mobility-assistive technology has multiple roles. Besides providing home and community accessibility, it plays a role in the child's overall development. These devices facilitate learning and social development. These devices also need to be tailored to the child's developmental needs. Failure to provide access to the appropriate devices limits children's ability to achieve their full potential.[1]

Butler[2] published a case series of 8 children mostly with spinal muscular atrophy (SMA) type II. The youngest child who was able to achieve safe and independent power mobility was 24 months old. One child began learning the task of operating a powered mobility device at 20 months of age. These children were all of normal intelligence.[1] Common diagnoses considered for early power mobility include SMA type II, congenital muscular dystrophies, congenital myopathies, congenital myasthenic syndromes, and Charcot-Marie-Tooth (CMT) type 3 or Dejerine-Sottas disease. Butler and colleagues[2] subsequently studied the effects of powered mobility on the development of young children with locomotor disability. They showed that learning powered mobility at 24 months had benefits on the frequency of self-initiated interaction with objects, spatial exploration, and communication with caregivers.

MANUAL WHEELCHAIRS

Patients with milder or more slowly progressive NMD can often use a manual wheelchair as their primary mode of mobility. Decreased exercise tolerance either caused by primary muscle or cardiopulmonary effects of the disease needs to be taken into consideration in determining what type of manual wheelchair would be most appropriate.

Manual wheelchairs can be divided into independent versus dependent devices. Independent manual wheelchairs (eg, lightweight or ultralightweight manual wheelchairs) can be used early in the disease to provide some level of energy conservation for community mobility for patients who may be able to ambulate only household distances.[3] Dependent manual wheelchairs (eg, tilt-in-space manual wheelchairs) may become necessary as the disease progresses and patients are no longer able to perform any type of independent mobility or cognitive dysfunction limits their ability to use forms of independent mobility. Dependent manual wheelchairs are pushed by the caregiver. Dependent-type wheelchairs, although heavier, can better accommodate additional devices such as adaptive communication devices, ventilators, and feeding pumps. These types of wheelchairs can serve as a backup manual wheelchair for primary power wheelchair users.

A manual wheelchair should be ordered early during the disease process to be used as a community mobility device for household ambulators that may require a mobility device for community mobility. Obtaining a manual wheelchair that can later serve as a backup chair when powered mobility is initiated should be considered if powered mobility is anticipated in the future. The subsequent power wheelchair is approved because of medical necessity caused by the disease progression. It is important to have a backup form of mobility in case of emergencies when access to electricity is limited or absent.

GEARED AND POWER-ASSIST WHEELCHAIRS AND MOBILITY DEVICES

Power-assist and geared devices are more appropriate for those who have a more slowly progressive disease. These devices can be adjusted to reduce the physical effort and endurance required to self-propel. Since the power-assist devices are attached to a manual wheelchair frame, they are lighter and more portable than a traditional power wheelchair. Some patients may choose this option to try to reduce the stigma of being in a larger power wheelchair. Others use these devices because they have suboptimal proximal shoulder girdle strength to propel standard wheelchairs for long distances. Power-assist wheels or rims (**Fig. 1**) have an electrical motor attached to the wheel. The rim senses the push and turns the wheel at an accelerated rate. These wheels can be interchanged with traditional wheels.

Geared devices use mechanical means to reduce the force required to propel a wheelchair. They allows the user to modify the gearing of either levers or the hand rim to propel the wheel at a different ratio than a standard hand rim. They can be considered if an individual lives or works in an area where access to electricity for long periods of time is limited. Users often interchange them with standard hand rims when needed.

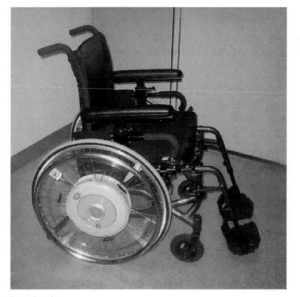

Fig. 1. Power-assist wheels.

SCOOTERS

Power Scooters can be a good option for patients who are in a transition period between ambulation and full-time wheelchair use. They can also be used for more slowly progressive diseases in which fatigue is one of the major symptoms. Patients who use scooters must have good arm strength, trunk balance, and core strength to transition in and out of the scooter. Patients with progressive disease processes that start more distally, such as hereditary sensory motor neuropathy or slowly progressive distal myopathies, may be good candidates for scooters. For ambulators, scooters are also easier to transfer to and from because of the relatively elevated seat height in comparison with a standard wheelchair. In addition, the seats often rotate 90° to facilitate transitions from sitting to standing.

POWER-ASSISTIVE MOBILITY DEVICES

Power mobility is the primary mode of mobility for many patients with NMD, especially at the later stages of a disease process. Power mobility requires the least strength. Patients who may be dependent for most activities of daily living are still capable of independent mobility. Power mobility must also be considered for patients in whom fatigue and lack of endurance are significant components of the disease process.[3] Energy conservation allows patients to be able to focus more on activities of daily living and vocational activities instead of exhausting all energy for mobility.

Complex power wheelchairs are commonly used in neuromuscular disorders. A complex power wheelchair is modifiable in virtually every aspect including the seating system, accessories such as armrests and headrests, as well as the control interface and switches. Some models have a seat-to-floor mode option so that children can participate in age-appropriate floor activities (**Fig. 2**). It also allows increased independence for those individuals who have the strength to perform floor-to-seat transfers. Power chairs can be made to accommodate other devices, such as a tray for mounting a mechanical ventilator or biphasic positive airway pressure machine.

Control Interfaces

There are various input options for controlling power mobility. For proportion control inputs such as a movement-sensing joystick (MSJ), the speed and direction of the chair depends on how far away from the center and in what direction the joystick is

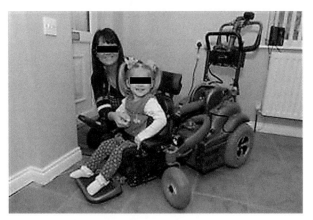

Fig. 2. Child with SMA II with a seat-to-floor mode.

pushed. MSJs can be programmed to accommodate ataxias by varying the sensitivity of the joystick. For significant weakness, the joystick can be programmed to require less travel for the same output. Additional hand-operated control input options include trackpads, which are similar to laptop mousepads and register a direction and velocity based on the movement of the finger touch away from a neutral center. An accelerometer head array registers the proportional distance of the head from the neutral upright position to determine the speed and direction of the powered mobility device. Force-sensing joysticks (FSJs) are another type of proportional control that uses a fixed joystick with force sensors to create a proportional output. The joystick operates as a proportional control just like an MSJ; however, the FSJ does not move when a force is applied. FSJs can be effective for patients with ataxia or tremors because they can provide stabilization to reduce excessive movement.[4,5]

Nonproportional control systems include the sip-and-puff system and head array system. The sip-and-puff system uses a breath tube that registers pressures to differentiate between hard and soft sips and puffs provided by the pressure in the patient's mouth so it can be used in patients with significant limb weakness with preserved breath support. The different patterns are then programmed to perform various functions for the powered mobility device. The head array system is a 3-piece headrest with switch pads in posterior and lateral positions, which the user activates by head movement. The controller is programmed to provide different functions based on the switch activation timing. For example, on a head array system, the user can access different menus to change speed, activate seat functions, or activate external environmental controls solely through the head array switches. Access to speed change menus also helps minimize lack of proportionality through the head array.

SEATING AND POSITIONING

Seating and positioning affect function and the ability to perform activities of daily living. The goals of the patient and caregivers need to be assessed by an experienced seating team. In NMD, seating systems need to take into account disease progression. The clinician needs to consider the timing of surgical correction such as spine fusion or tendon lengthening because this affects seating and positioning. There are multiple options for seating and positioning from headrest to footrest. Some of these options are easily modifiable for disease progression.

Headrests

Headrests support the head and neck when there is decreased head and neck control. Patients with weak neck extensors, such as those with SMA, Duchenne muscular dystrophy (DMD), congenital muscular dystrophies, or amyotrophic lateral sclerosis (ALS), may require anterior or lateral head supports such as a headband or an anterior forehead pad. Swallow function must be taken into consideration during placement of anterior headrests. Some patients require more cervical flexion while eating to reduce the risk of aspiration.

Seat Backs

There are various types of seat backs, from a fabric sling backrest to a custom-molded back support. Scoliosis is a common complication of severe pediatric NMDs. To accommodate either a fixed or flexible spinal deformity, lateral supports, anterior trunk supports, and armrest position need to be considered. Custom-contoured seat backs can accommodate more severe deformities. Custom-contoured seat backs tend to be less adjustable and do not allow for movement within the seat. Proper trunk support also affects how pressure is distributed on the seat cushion, which is important for prevention of skin breakdown.

Recline and Seat Back Angle

The seat-to-back angle or recline of the seating system can either be fixed, manually adjustable, or powered. When the seat-to-back angle is changed frequently, there is a tendency for the patient to slide out of the chair. Many manufacturers have tried to correct this problem by developing low-shear backrests that slide up and down with the patient's back. Benefits of power recline include aiding activities of daily living such as voiding in a urinal.[6]

Seat Elevator

A power seat elevator should be considered for patients with limited upper extremity active range of motion (**Fig. 3**). The seat elevator allows patients to reach higher items or to work in environments in which counters or tables may not be at a traditional wheelchair level. A seat elevator can also be an important tool in independent transfers for those with proximal weakness. It can also reduce the caregiver burden of a patient who requires dependent transfers.[7]

Wheelchair Cushions

The primary function of a wheelchair cushion is to mitigate the effects of pressure on the bony prominences of the sitting surface. The relief of pressure also translates to improved sitting comfort. It is important to take into account the pressure-distributing properties of the cushions in relation to the overall seating system because patients

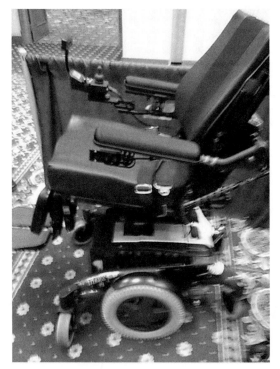

Fig. 3. Power seat elevator.

with progressive NMD have limited mobility. In general, as pressure relieving properties increase, the stability of the seating surface decreases. The primary materials can be broken down into 2 groups: foam and fluids (which includes air and gel).

Foam is the most common material found in cushions. It deforms in proportion depending on both the stiffness and thickness of the material. The foam material is elastic and thus constantly exerts a force to return to its unloaded state. In areas where the foam deforms the most, such as below the ischial tuberosity, the foam may cause enough pressure to cause ischemia to the skin, increasing risk for pressure sores. Foam provides the most stability for patients with decreased sitting balance.

Air has low viscous properties that readily equalize pressure within a container. Air is generally contained in either an elastic rubber or plastic base material. These materials have elastic properties that mitigate effects on the ability of air to equalize pressure on sitting surfaces. Gel is a fluid that also equalizes pressure, depending on the viscosity. Often air or gel is used in combination with a foam base. Air or gel is placed to equalize pressure from the bony prominence of the pelvis. The foam base provides a more stable sitting surface than air or gel alone.

Custom-contoured cushions restrict movement of the sitting surface but can provide a stable surface to improve range of active distal movement. They can accommodate significant orthopedic deformity related to disease progression, such as an increased pelvic obliquity associated with a progressive scoliosis. Many patients with intact sensation, as is the case with most NMDs, do not find custom-contoured cushions comfortable because of the restricted movement.

Two additional subsets of specialized wheelchair seating include force isolation seats and alternating pressure. Force isolation seats borrow from orthotic principles of transferring pressure. These seats are shaped to transfer pressure from high-risk areas such as the greater trochanters and ischial tuberosities to areas that are more tolerant of pressure, such as the distal and proximal thigh and gluteal areas. Alternating pressure cushions use an electric pump to fill alternating bladders, allowing blood flow to skin where the localized bladder was deflated. This type of cushion can result in instability; however, it is a solution for patients who have refractory skin breakdown using alternative cushions.

Leg Rest

Leg rests can either be fixed or elevating. The method of elevating the leg rest can be either manual or power. Dependent edema is a common problem in patients with lower limb weakness caused by the lack of limb muscle contractions aiding in venous return. Often there is purplish discoloration of the lower extremities and edema can cause discomfort. The ability to raise the legs helps to reduce the edema and improves comfort by improving venous return. In addition, elevating leg rests can also help prevent or reduce progressive knee flexion contractures that can result in positioning difficulties, especially when supine in bed. Elevating leg rests can also provide pressure relief off the cushion.[8]

Footrests

Footrests are generally chosen to accommodate contractures associated with NMD. In DMD, equinus contractures are common and angle adjustable foot rests are ideal to accommodate contractures.[9] Cushioned foot rests made of similar materials used in pressure relieving seat cushions are used when foot and ankle contractures are severe. The cushioned foot rests improve comfort and reduce the risk for pressure sores on the feet and ankles.

AUGMENTATIVE ALTERNATIVE COMMUNICATION AND ENVIRONMENTAL CONTROLS

There are various ways in which patients with significant motor impairment can use assistive technology to interact with their community and environment. The wheelchair can serve either as a mechanical or electronic platform for assistive technology devices. Augmentative communication and environmental control devices can all be directly mounted on a wheelchair for ease of access using trays or swing-away post mounts. Home appliances can be modified so that they can be directly accessed from a wheelchair.

There are several different types of augmentative communication devices and programs. These devices are recommended for patients who are not able to produce intelligible vocalizations. Augmentative communication may be as simple as pointing to pictures or photographs. More complicated devices include computers requiring the user to either type the word or pull together pictures to form a sentence that is then verbalized using a synthetic text-to-speech output. There are multiple alternative ways to control augmentative communication devices.[4]

Keyboards

Keyboards or tablet computers can be mounted on a wheelchair tray. The keys on the keyboard can be modified depending on the motor control or cognition level of the patient. The keys can be expanded to accommodate excessive movement, as seen in Friedreich ataxia. Keyboards can have different key layouts rather than the traditional QWERTY keyboard. They can also be smaller for those with minimal active movement of the fingers.[4]

Scanning Systems

For patients with significant motor impairments such as SMA I, congenital muscular dystrophies, or late stages of ALS and DMD, a scanning system can be implemented. A program automatically scrolls through a selection of menus or choices. Once the menu or choice has been highlighted by the program, the user activates various types of switches to activate that selection.[4,7]

Remote Environmental Controls

In general, a chair that requires alternative controls and has a display also has the capability for infrared and Bluetooth interface with other technologies. Through infrared output, the joystick can mimic the use of a remote control for a television set, stereo system, door openers, and light switches. Through the Bluetooth connection, the display and joystick can be set up to operate a computer using the power chair controls as a mouse input. The joystick can be equipped with a juxtaposed mouse emulator with right and left mouse buttons alongside the joystick (**Fig. 4**). The joystick can be toggled into a mode in which, through a Bluetooth interface, it can be used as a computer mouse. These interfaces are essential for patients who do not have access or do not want to rely on caregivers for these tasks. They are also essential for patients who use computer technology as their primary vocation.

Voice Recognition

Voice recognition software can be an option for those with limited upper limb function to interface with environmental and wheelchair controls.[4] The application of this technology is limited by the decreased vital capacity and need for daytime ventilation that is often seen in patients with the degree of paralysis necessitating the use of the voice

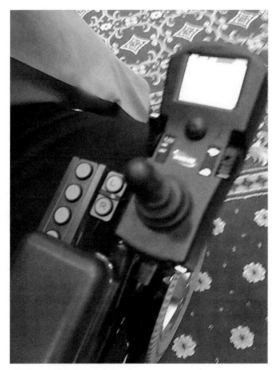

Fig. 4. Joystick as wireless mouse emulator.

recognition technology. For these patients, the scanning interfaces can be more functional.

Eye Gaze

Eye gaze sensing technology is an effective and consistent method for accessing augmentative communication devices and environmental control systems. The eye gaze system senses movement from the reflection of the eye. It can be used in any position either in the bed or the wheelchair. Eye gaze technology continues to improve and it provides access to communication and the environment and increased hope for people at the later stages of progressive NMD.

Brain Computer Interface

Brain computer interface is an emerging method of activation of mobility devices and environmental controls. Electrocorticography involves inserting cortical microelectrodes to pick up cortical signals. The signals are filtered through a computer to perform a specific task. Patients have been able to control cursors using signals from electrocorticography for short periods of time. This signal has not been attempted to control a device in 3 dimensions. Electroencephalography is a less invasive approach because electrodes are placed on the scalp. Attempts have been made to use electroencephalography signals, but the information obtained has been limited because of the filtering properties of the skull.[10]

SUMMARY

Mobility-assistive technologies allow patients with NMD to interact with peers and with the community. In children, they also serve to facilitate development, and lack of access to the appropriate devices can have adverse developmental consequences. Children with severe weakness and intact cognition should begin to be fit for power wheelchairs before their second birthday. There are multiple options for mobility devices and methods for their control. These devices can be integrated with other electronics to facilitate the control of a variety of devices in the environment. The clinician must be aware of the natural history of progressive NMDs and anticipate the need for modifications to the assistive mobility device.

REFERENCES

1. Butler C, Okamoto GA, McKay TM. Powered mobility for very young disabled children. Dev Med Child Neurol 1983;25(4):472–4.
2. Butler C. Effects of powered mobility on self-initiated behaviors of very young children with locomotor disability. Dev Med Child Neurol 1986;28(3):325–32.
3. Souza A, Kelleher A, Cooper R, et al. Multiple sclerosis and mobility-related assistive technology: systematic review of literature. J Rehabil Res Dev 2010; 47(3):213–23.
4. Braddom RL. Physical medicine and rehabilitation. 4th edition. Philadelphia: WB Saunders; 2011.
5. Dicianno BE, Cooper RA, Coltellaro J. Joystick control for powered mobility: current state of technology and future directions. Phys Med Rehabil Clin North Am 2010;21(1):79–86.
6. Liu M, Mineo K, Hanayama K, et al. Practical problems and management of seating through the clinical stages of Duchenne's muscular dystrophy. Arch Phys Med Rehabil 2003;84(6):818–24.
7. Cooper RA, Cooper R. Quality-of-life technology for people with spinal cord injuries. Phys Med Rehabil Clin North Am 2010;21(1):1–13.
8. Aissaoui R, Heydar S, Dansereau J, et al. Biomechanical analysis of legrest support of occupied wheelchairs: comparison between a conventional and a compensatory legrest. IEEE Trans Rehabil Eng 2000;8(1):140–8.
9. McDonald CM, Abresch RT, Carter GT, et al. Profiles of neuromuscular diseases. Duchenne muscular dystrophy. Am J Phys Med Rehabil 1995;74(Suppl 5): S70–92.
10. Cooper RA, Dicianno BE, Brewer B, et al. A perspective on intelligent devices and environments in medical rehabilitation. Med Eng Phys 2008;30(10):1387–98.

Chronic Pain in Neuromuscular Disease

Pain Site and Intensity Differentially Impacts Function

Jordi Miró, PhD[a], Kevin J. Gertz, PhD[b],
Gregory T. Carter, MD, MS[c,d,e],*, Mark P. Jensen, PhD[b]

KEYWORDS

- Neuromuscular disease • Chronic pain • Pain intensity • Muscular dystrophy
- Regional pain

KEY POINTS

- Most patients with slowly progressive neuromuscular disease have chronic pain, to some degree. The studies done to date have typically assessed average pain intensity rather than occurrence and severity of pain in specific body locations. This assessment limits the usefulness of the data with respect to formulating treatment plans that address both physical and psychological aspects of pain.
- The available data suggest that pain extent and intensity at specific sites are associated with pain interference and negatively affect both physical and psychological functioning in patients with slowly progressive neuromuscular disease.
- Future studies assessing pain in persons with slowly progressive neuromuscular disease should address pain site in addition to global pain intensity. Investigating pain at multiple sites in future studies will enable clinicians to design more effective therapeutic interventions to treat pain in this patient population.

INTRODUCTION

A growing body of research indicates that chronic pain is a significant problem for many persons with chronic, slowly progressive neuromuscular disease (NMD).[1–16]

[a] Unit for the Study and Treatment of Pain - ALGOS, Centre de Recerca en Avaluació i Mesura del Comportament, Institut d'Investigació Sanitària Pere Virgili, Universitat Rovira i Virgili, Carretera de Valls s7N, 43007 Tarragona, Catalonia, Spain; [b] Department of Rehabilitation Medicine, University of Washington School of Medicine, Box 359612, Seattle, WA 98195, USA; [c] Department of Clinical Neurosciences, Providence Medical Group, Olympia, WA 98506, USA; [d] Department of Physical Medicine and Rehabilitation, University of California at Davis, Sacramento, CA 95817, USA; [e] MEDEX Division, University of Washington School of Medicine, Seattle, WA 98195, USA
* Corresponding author. PO Box 1019, Centralia, WA 98531.
E-mail address: gtcarter@uw.edu

Phys Med Rehabil Clin N Am 23 (2012) 895–902
http://dx.doi.org/10.1016/j.pmr.2012.08.008
1047-9651/12/$ – see front matter © 2012 Elsevier Inc. All rights reserved.

However, it is still not clear how much pain intensity factors in to the negative bio-psychosocial and physical consequences of chronic pain in the setting of slowly progressive NMD. Pain intensity is one of the most common dimensions assessed by clinicians and researchers who treat and study pain. Reduction in global pain intensity is also the standard by which most pain treatments are judged. However, although average pain intensity is an important pain domain, other pain domains are also potentially important (eg, pain frequency, duration, location, and quality) as factors that could contribute to patient dysfunction, especially in individuals with chronic pain.[17] Unfortunately, research is lacking regarding the relative importance of these additional domains for understanding adjustment to pain.

The research that has been conducted on this topic in other pain populations suggests that pain site may contribute to adjustment to chronic pain over and above the effects of global pain intensity. For example, Marshall and colleagues[18] found that the intensity of back pain in patients with amputation explained a significant amount of variance in interference in daily activities beyond the pain associated with limb amputation. Similarly, there is some preliminary evidence that pain in the low back and arms is more strongly associated with patient functioning than pain in other body locations in a sample of patients with a variety of chronic pain problems (Tan G, Jensen MP, unpublished data, 2011). Nonetheless, research in this area is sparse, and it is not known whether these preliminary findings replicate in other samples of patients with chronic pain, including those with NMD. If these findings do replicate across different chronic pain populations, then clinicians should assess both pain intensity and its location(s) to better understand the potential impact that the pain might have on a specific patient. Moreover, if low back pain or pain in the extremities is more closely linked to a patient's quality of life than pain at other sites, then treatments that address pain at these sites may be more important to patients with chronic pain than treatments that address pain at other sites (eg, the head or torso). Thus, research in this area could help inform the work of clinicians and scientists who are developing new pain treatments for individuals with specific pain conditions. However, the authors are not aware of any research that has studied the relative importance of pain site to patient functioning in individuals with slowly progressive NMD.

Pain extent is a separate and distinct domain from intensity and refers to the overall number of body areas with pain. Research suggests that this pain domain may also be important to patient functioning. For example, Tait and colleagues[19] found a significant association between pain extent and the tendency of patients to report greater complaints of weakness, fatigue, and depression. Similarly, Toomey and colleagues[20] reported that patients with more pain sites were more likely to report pain as having a greater negative impact in their functioning. Türp and colleagues[21] found that pain extent, along with pain intensity, was a significant predictor of pain-related disability in a sample of female patients with chronic facial pain. Patients with pain at multiple sites have shown a reduced level of health-related functioning, are more likely to have difficulties with mobility regardless of physical impairments than those with no pain or localized pain, and have worse prognosis for future work ability.[22–24] In a series of studies, Kamaleri and colleagues[25] reported significant associations between pain extent and functioning in patients with musculoskeletal pain. They found a strong and linear association between increasing number of pain sites and decreasing functional ability; a strong relationship with decreasing psychological health, sleep quality, and overall health; and future work disability after a 14-year period.[25,26]

As with research on the importance of specific pain sites to patient functioning, it is unclear if these findings regarding pain extent replicate in other populations of individuals with chronic pain, including persons with slowly progressive NMD. Most published studies on these issues have been conducted with low back patients receiving treatment at secondary and tertiary care facilities. Thus, these findings may not generalize to other populations of patients with pain.[27]

Further delineating the relative importance of pain site and extent in relation to patient functioning is particularly important in patients with NMD, because research indicates they typically experience pain in more than one location.[5] Given what previous studies have found in other pain populations, the authors hypothesize that pain extent would be negatively associated with psychological functioning and positively associated with pain interference, whereas pain intensity in specific pain sites would show stronger associations with measures of patient functioning than pain at other sites. More specifically, one would expect that pain in the low back and arms might evidence stronger associations with pain interference and psychological functioning than pain at other sites.

DISEASE-SPECIFIC PAIN TRAITS

There are intriguing differences among degrees of pain in the slowly progressive forms of NMD. It is not unexpected that neuropathic diseases like Charcot Marie Tooth would rank high in pain intensity, given the pathogenesis of the disease, particularly the demyelinating forms. However, it is clear that 2 of the most common forms muscular dystrophy, myotonic type 1 (DM1), and facioscapulohumeral (FSHD), are also high on the list of painful NMDs.[5] Worldwide, DM1 and FSHD are the first and third most common forms of dystrophic myopathies, respectively, with the dystrophinopathies coming in second.[28] Both DM1 and FSHD are autosomal dominant, slowly progressive neuromuscular disorders (NMDs).[29,30] DM1 is caused by a polynucleotide (CTG) triplet expansion located on the 3′ untranslated region of chromosome 19q13.3.[31] This location results in a toxic gain of function of abnormally stored RNA in the nuclei of affected cells, leading to deregulation of RNA binding protein levels and mRNA splicing processes of multiple genes.[32,33] This action is presumed responsible for the multisystem features typical of DM1, with involvement of skeletal, cardiac, and smooth muscles, and the central nervous, endocrine, ocular, respiratory, and gastrointestinal systems to varying degrees.[34]

In FSHD, most patients possess a large deletion in the polymorphic D4Z4 macrosatellite repeat array at 4q35, presenting with up to 10 repeats, as opposed to 11–150 repeats in unaffected individuals.[35–37] This situation is complicated by a nearly identical repeat array present at 10q26.[34] The remarkably similar sequence identity between these 2 arrays can cause difficulties in molecular diagnosis. Each 3.3-kb D4Z4 unit contains a DUX4 (double homeobox 4) gene that is activated on contraction of the 4q35 repeat array via induction of chromatin remodeling.[36] Myofiber synthesis of both DUX4 transcripts and protein causes significant cell toxicity. As a transcription factor, DUX4 may target several genes, resulting in cellular deregulation with inhibition of myogenesis, muscle degradation, and oxidative stress.[35]

Prior studies indicate that as many as nearly 90% and 70% of patients with FSHD and DM1 report pain, respectively.[5,38,39] In addition to indentifying pain as a major problem for patients with either of these NDMs, these studies also indicate that pain is more common in patients with FSHD versus DM1.[1,5,9] The average severity of pain in patients with FSHD (approximately 4.4 of 10 on an ordinal pain scale) is less than that reported by patients with DM1 (6.28 of 10).[5] The reasons these disease in particular have more pain are not clear but they involve membrane-related pathology, and both disorders have underlying genetic expansion-type mutations and are multisystem disorders.[40]

As already mentioned, almost all previously published studies on the effects of pain extent have been conducted on patients with musculoskeletal problems. Results from these reports seem to support that simply counting the number of pain sites might be important when assessing a patient's pain problem.[41] This approach does not seem adequate, however, for people with an NMD. At least, for this specific population, our data suggest that overlooking the pain intensity of the specific sites may result in a failure to capture the true meaning and implications of the pain experience of these patients. Reasons for this failure include the fact that NMDs involve pathophysiology in the peripheral nerves or muscles as part of the underlying disease process, which is distinctly different from a musculoskeletal disorder. Thus, a variety of abnormal processes may generate and maintain the symptom of pain in NMDs, and conceptually, it is likely that no one mechanism may be disease specific, although this topic remains to be studied. It is more likely that any given NMD would have several mechanisms associated with it. Thus, accounting for the pain in any single patient may require hypothesizing one or more mechanisms at work simultaneously. Once neuropathic pain is present, all levels of the nervous system, peripheral, central, and autonomic, may play a role in the generation and maintenance of pain.[42–44] Therefore, independent of actual clinical diagnosis, several different pathophysiologic processes may be present simultaneously. Further, some patients with neuropathic pain may also develop secondary myofascial pain. Myofascial pain may mimic neuropathic pain and result in referred pain distant from the actual soft tissue source and is a logical explanation for the chain of events occurring in a hereditary neuropathy like Charcot Marie Tooth disease. However, these myofascial pain generators are likely further accentuated in diseased, dystrophic muscle such as seen in DM1 or FSHD.

It is probable that, to some extent, skeletal muscle pathophysiology plays a significant role in pain generation in this setting. Because of active, ongoing muscle degeneration, there is significant risk for overwork weakness and exercise-induced muscle injury, even with simply doing activities of daily living.[45] Dystrophic muscle is susceptible to exercise-induced muscle injury, particularly eccentric (lengthening) muscle contractions.[45] Patients with NMD are susceptible to overwork weakness and muscle injury, resulting in excessive delayed-onset muscle soreness. This soreness usually occurs 24–48 hours after exercise. Other symptoms might include muscle cramping, heaviness in the extremities, prolonged dyspnea, and fatigue. Fatigue in this setting is likely multifactorial because of deconditioning and impaired muscular activation, but likely contributes to pain.[46]

WHAT ARE THE NEXT STEPS?

The importance of considering pain site when assessing pain and its impact in persons with chronic pain is reinforced by data indicating that pain extent is significantly associated with pain interference and psychological functioning.[5,10] Pain extent likely plays a significant role in many chronic pain populations. The nature of pain in individuals with DM1 and FSHD suggests that this would be important in patients with these diagnoses as well. However, it is not clear whether pain in the low back and arms is more strongly associated with pain interference and psychological functioning than pain at other locations; research is needed to address this specific question. Nonetheless, the study findings reviewed support the idea that pain site matters, although further study is clearly warranted. It seems, however, that the pain sites that matter most to persons suffering from chronic pain in the setting of an NMD like DM1 or FSHD may differ significantly from those of persons with other chronic pain conditions.[47,48] The findings have important implications for understanding and treating, pain in persons with NMD.

Clearly, a comprehensive assessment of these persons will require going beyond the mere assessment of overall or general pain intensity and will require to gather information about the intensity of each pain problem. Thus, in this population, both a quantitative and qualitative assessment of the pain experience should be promoted. Especially relevant would be to attend to the pain in legs, feet, hips, and knees beyond overall pain intensity, because they are all significantly related to pain interference. Pain experienced in the head should also be addressed given its potential impact on psychological functioning above and beyond what is expected from overall pain intensity.

The authors also hypothesize that pain interference and psychological functioning are associated with pain intensity at different sites, although this hypothesis needs empiric confirmation with data. Intuitively, the sites most likely to exert the strongest (and unique) associations are the ones related to ambulation (ie, legs, feet, hips, and knees), which makes biomechanical sense, given that these muscles are particularly taxed physically and consequently susceptible to contraction-induced injury, as discussed earlier. Thus, it is important from a treatment perspective to address these individuals functionally, that is, devising specific strategies or activities to improve strength, flexibility, and endurance of those muscles and related areas. These areas are those that inflict higher interference and functioning tolls to the patients and should be addressed in any rehabilitation paradigm for these patients.

Turner and colleagues,[49] found that patients who reported more pain sites before participating in a cognitive-behavioral treatment had higher activity interference at 1 year; therefore, treatments for NMD patients should rely on pain intensity in specific sites rather than overall pain intensity ratings. Moreover, each pain site might require different approaches, with specific combinations of rehabilitation alternatives.

Our pilot study found that the "other" pain location significantly contributed to the variance of pain interference. It was just a small group of participants (N = 19) that reported experiencing pain in a location or locations other than those in the survey (Miró J, et al, 2012). However, there seem to be other location(s) that are important to explain pain interference in people with an NMD and chronic pain beyond those analyzed in this study. Future work might build on the findings of this study by attempting to determine other pain locations that might be of importance for these patients to address them when developing treatment programs.

Some important limitations to the available published literature should be considered when interpreting the results. Most patient samples primarily include patients registered with the national Institutes of Health–funded MD National Registry, and the extent to which the findings from these patients are broadly applicable to individuals with other forms of NMD is not known. Moreover, all information is usually based on self-report measures. Therefore, it is possible that some of the significant associations found between measures may, therefore, be related to shared method variance. Future researchers should examine the associations between pain at different sites and more objective measures of patient functioning, such as ratings made by spouses or significant others, or objective measures of activity (eg, actigraphy).

Despite limited data, the available studies provide support for the potential utility of assessing specific pain qualities and overall pain intensity measures in persons with slowly progressive NMD, hence, the need for more studies of the influence of pain site and extent in patients with slowly progressive NMDs. Further studies are needed to explore and confirm these complex interrelationships. Nevertheless, there seem to be enough data, both from chronic pain populations and from patients whose pain is secondary to a disability, to support the inclusion of pain quality characteristics as outcome variables in pain research.[18,22,25,26]

ACKNOWLEDGMENTS

This research was supported by the National Institutes of Health, National Institute of Child Health and Human Development, National Center for Rehabilitation Research (grant no. P01HD33988), the National Registry of Myotonic Dystrophy and Facioscapulohumeral Muscular Dystrophy Patients and Family Members, and the National Institute on Disability Rehabilitation Research (grant no. H133B031118). JM's work is supported by grants from the Government of Catalonia, AGAUR (Refs: 2009 SGR 434, and DGR 2011BE1 00611), and Vicerectorat de Recerca of Universitat Rovira i Virgili.

REFERENCES

1. Jensen MP, Moore MR, Bockow TB, et al. Psychosocial factors and adjustment to chronic pain in persons with physical disabilities: a systematic review. Arch Phys Med Rehabil 2011;92(1):146–60.
2. Jensen MP, Abresch RT, Carter GT, et al. Chronic pain in persons with neuromuscular disorders. Arch Phys Med Rehabil 2005;86(6):1155–63.
3. Suokas KI, Haanpää M, Kautiainen H, et al. Pain in patients with myotonic dystrophy type 2: a postal survey in Finland. Muscle Nerve 2012;45(1):70–4.
4. Abresch RT, Carter GT, Jensen MP, et al. Assessment of pain and health-related quality of life in slowly progressive neuromuscular disease. Am J Hosp Palliat Care 2002;19(1):39–48.
5. Jensen MP, Hoffman AJ, Stoelb BL, et al. Chronic pain in persons with myotonic and facioscapulohumeral muscular dystrophy. Arch Phys Med Rehabil 2008; 89(2):320–8.
6. Hirsch AT, Kupper AE, Carter GT, et al. Psychosocial factors and adjustment to pain in individuals with postpolio syndrome. Am J Phys Med Rehabil 2010; 89(3):213–24.
7. Molton I, Jensen MP, Ehde DM, et al. Coping with chronic pain among younger, middle-aged, and older adults living with neurologic injury and disease: a role for experiential wisdom. J Aging Health 2008;20:972–96.
8. Stoelb BL, Carter GT, Abresch RT, et al. Pain in persons with postpolio syndrome: frequency, intensity, and impact. Arch Phys Med Rehabil 2008;89(10):1933–40.
9. Carter GT, Jensen MP, Stoelb BL, et al. Chronic pain in persons with myotonic muscular dystrophy, type 1. Arch Phys Med Rehabil 2008;89(12):2382.
10. Nieto R, Raichle KA, Jensen MP, et al. Changes in pain-related beliefs, coping, and catastrophizing predict changes in pain intensity, pain interference, and psychological functioning in individuals with myotonic muscular dystrophy and facioscapulohumeral dystrophy. Clin J Pain 2012;28(1):47–54.
11. Engel JM, Kartin D, Carter GT, et al. Pain in youths with neuromuscular disease. Am J Hosp Palliat Care 2009;26(5):405–12.
12. Engel JM, Kartin D, Jaffe KM. Exploring chronic pain in youths with Duchenne Muscular Dystrophy: a model for pediatric neuromuscular disease. Phys Med Rehabil Clin N Am 2005;16(4):1113–24.
13. Miró J, Raichle KA, Carter GT, et al. Impact of biopsychosocial factors on chronic pain in persons with myotonic and facioscapulohumeral muscular dystrophy. Am J Hosp Palliat Care 2009;26(4):308–19.
14. Carter GT, Jensen MP, Galer BS, et al. Neuropathic pain in Charcot Marie Tooth disease. Arch Phys Med Rehabil 1998;79:1560–4.
15. Abresch RT, Jensen MP, Carter GT. Health quality of life in peripheral neuropathy. Phys Med Rehabil Clin N Am 2001;12(2):461–72.

16. Hoffman AJ, Jensen MP, Abresch RT, et al. Chronic pain in persons with neuro-muscular disorders. Phys Med Rehabil Clin N Am 2005;16(4):1099–112.
17. Von Korff M, Dunn KM. Chronic pain reconsidered. Pain 2008;138:267–76.
18. Marshall HM, Jensen MP, Ehde DM, et al. Pain site and impairment in individuals with amputation pain. Arch Phys Med Rehabil 2002;83:1116–9.
19. Tait RC, Chibnall JT, Margolis RB. Pain extent: relations with psychological state, pain severity, pain history, and disability. Pain 1990;41:295–301.
20. Toomey TC, Mann JD, Abashian S, et al. Relationship of pain drawing scores to ratings of pain description and function. Clin J Pain 1991;7:269–74.
21. Türp C, Kowalski CJ, Stohler CS. Greater disability with increased pain involve-ment, pain intensity and depressive preoccupation. Eur J Pain 1997;1:271–7.
22. Saastamoinen P, Leino-Arjas P, Laaksonen M, et al. Pain and health related func-tioning among employees. J Epidemiol Community Health 2006;60:793–8.
23. Leveille SG, Bean J, Ngo L, et al. The pathway from musculoskeletal pain to mobility difficulty in older disabled women. Pain 2007;128:69–77.
24. Natvig B, Eriksen W, Bruusgaard D. Low back pain as a predictor of long-term work disability. Scand J Public Health 2002;30:288–92.
25. Kamaleri Y, Natvig B, Ihlebaek CM, et al. Localized or widespread musculoskel-etal pain: does it matter? Pain 2008;138:41–6.
26. Kamaleri Y, Natvig B, Ihlebaek CM, et al. Does the number of musculoskeletal pain sites predict work disability? A 14-year predictive study. Eur J Pain 2009; 13:426–30.
27. Carnes D, Parsons S, Ashby D, et al. Chronic musculoskeletal pain rarely pres-ents in a single body site: results from a UK population study. Rheumatology 2007;46:1168–70.
28. Emery AH. Population frequencies of inherited neuromuscular diseases. A world survey. Neuromuscul Disord 1991;1:19–25.
29. Kilmer DD, Abresch RT, Aitkens SG, et al. Profiles of neuromuscular disease: facioscapulohumeral dystrophy. Am J Phys Med Rehabil 1995;74(5):S131–9.
30. Johnson ER, Carter GT, Kilmer DD, et al. Profiles of neuromuscular disease: myotonic muscular dystrophy. Am J Phys Med Rehabil 1995;74(5):S104–16.
31. Ashizawa T, Dubel JR, Dunne PW, et al. Anticipation in myotonic dystrophy: II. complex relationships between clinical findings and structure of the GCT repeat. Neurology 1992;42:1877–81.
32. Redman JB, Fenwick RG, Fu Y, et al. Relationship between parental trinucleotide GCT repeat length and severity of myotonic dystrophy in offspring. JAMA 1993; 269:1960–72.
33. Hunter A, Tsilfidis C, Mettler G, et al. The correlation of age of onset with CTG trinucleotide repeat amplification in myotonic dystrophy. J Med Genet 1992;29: 774–81.
34. Harley H, Rundle SA, MacMillan JC, et al. Size of the unstable CTG repeat sequence in relation to phenotype and parental transmission in myotonic dystrophy. Am J Hum Genet 1993;52:1164–71.
35. Wijmenga C, Frants RR, Brouwer OF, et al. The facioscapulohumeral muscular dystrophy gene maps to chromosome 4. Lancet 1990;2:651–8.
36. Upadhyaya M, Lunt PW, Sarfarazi M, et al. DNA marker applicable to presymp-tomatic and prenatal diagnosis of facioscapulohumeral disease. Lancet 1990; 336:1320–7.
37. Snider L, Geng LN, Lemmers RJ, et al. Facioscapulohumeral dystrophy: incomplete suppression of a retrotransposed gene. PLoS Genet 2010;6(10): e1001181.

38. Bushby KM, Pollitt C, Johnson MA, et al. Muscle pain as a prominent feature of facioscapulohumeral muscular dystrophy (FSHD): four illustrative case reports. Neuromuscul Disord 1998;8:574–9.

39. Kalkman JS, Schillings ML, van der Werf SP, et al. Experienced fatigue in facioscapulohumeral dystrophy, myotonic dystrophy, and HMSN-I. J Neurol Neurosurg Psychiatry 2005;76(10):1406–9.

40. Verhagen WI, Huygen PL, Padberg GW. The auditory, vestibular and oculomotor system in facioscapulohumeral dystrophy. Acta Otolaryngol 1995;1:140–52.

41. Schmidt CO, Baumeister SE. Simple patterns behind complex spatial pain reporting? Assessing a classification of multisite pain reporting in the general population. Pain 2007;133:174–82.

42. Pazzaglia C, Vollono C, Ferraro D, et al. Mechanisms of neuropathic pain in patients with Charcot-Marie-Tooth 1 A: a laser-evoked potential study. Pain 2010;149(2):379–85.

43. Ribiere C, Bernardin M, Sacconi S, et al. Pain assessment in Charcot-Marie-Tooth (CMT) disease. Ann Phys Rehabil Med 2012;55(3):160–73.

44. Padua L, Cavallaro T, Pareyson D, et al. Italian CMT QoL Study Group. Charcot-Marie-Tooth and pain: correlations with neurophysiological, clinical, and disability findings. Neurol Sci 2008;29(3):193–4.

45. Abresch RT, Han JJ, Carter GT. Rehabilitation management of neuromuscular disease: the role of exercise training. J Clin Neuromuscul Dis 2009;11(1):7–21.

46. Lou JS, Weiss MD, Carter GT. Assessment and management of fatigue in neuromuscular disease. Am J Hosp Palliat Care 2010;27(2):145–57.

47. Tiffreau V, Viet G, Thévenon A. Pain and neuromuscular disease: the results of a survey. Am J Phys Med Rehabil 2006;85(9):756–66.

48. Guy-Coichard C, Nguyen DT, Delorme T, et al. Pain in hereditary neuromuscular disorders and myasthenia gravis: a national survey of frequency, characteristics, and impact. J Pain Symptom Manage 2008;35(1):40–50.

49. Turner JA, Holtzman S, Mancl L. Mediators, moderators, and predictors of therapeutic change in cognitive-behavioral therapy for chronic pain. Pain 2007;127:276–86.

Using Palliative Care in Progressive Neuromuscular Disease to Maximize Quality of Life

Gregory T. Carter, MD, MS[a,b,]*, Nanette C. Joyce, DO[a], Allison L. Abresch, DO[c], Amanda E. Smith, BS[d], Gregg K. VandeKeift, MD, MA[b]

KEYWORDS

- Neuromuscular disease • Palliative care • Chronic pain • Burden of disease
- Quality of life • Muscular dystrophy

KEY POINTS

- Palliative medical care is a new subspecialty in medicine, emerging in the past decade.
- People with severe neuromuscular diseases (NMDs), like Duchenne muscular dystrophy (DMD), are now living well in to adulthood, making them a previously unseen, unstudied population of patients.
- These 2 new entities—"palliative care" and "adults with DMD," or any NMD patient who is living with an advanced form of NMD—would seem ideally suited for each other.
- Palliative care strategies are optimal to alleviate suffering in patients with an advanced NMD because they target the complexity of symptoms seen in this population.
- There is a great need for more research in patients with NMD who are receiving palliative services to create best practice standards in pain and symptom management for this population.

INTRODUCTION

Defining Palliative Care

Palliative care is a relatively new medical subspecialty, having arisen from a necessity for improved ways to manage patients with chronic diseases that may be

This research was supported by the National Institute for Disability Rehabilitation Research (grant H133B0900001). The authors have nothing to disclose.

[a] Department of Physical Medicine and Rehabilitation, University of California at Davis, 2315 Stockton Boulevard, Sacramento, CA 95817, USA; [b] Hospice and Palliative Care Services, Providence Health Services, 413 Lilly Road Northeast, Olympia, WA 98506-5166, USA; [c] Department of Family Medicine, Good Samaritan Hospital, 3600 NW Samaritan Drive, Corvallis, OR 97330, USA; [d] Department of Rehabilitation Medicine, University of Washington School of Medicine, Box 356490, Seattle, WA 98195, USA
* Corresponding author. PO Box 1019, Centralia, WA 98531.
E-mail address: gtcarter@uw.edu

"life-limiting." Palliative care is similar in some ways to hospice care, yet it has enough distinct features to emerge as a sovereign entity. In fact, palliative care requires a paradigm shift away from the "hospice mindset," in which death is a forthcoming and soon expected outcome (or "death is expected within 6 months"). This is not the case in palliative care, in which patients may seek similarly aggressive treatment of their symptoms, including pain, at any time during the disease course, for which death may not occur for many years. Here, successful management warrants more frequent patient reassessments and significant pharmacovigilance.

Despite similarity in the philosophy of care and services rendered, in the US health care system, palliative care and hospice services have 2 different payment systems and locations of services.[1,2] Hospice is the only Medicare benefit that includes pharmaceuticals, medical equipment, 24-hours-a-day/7-days-a-week access to care, and support for loved ones following a death. Most hospice care is delivered at home, but it is also available to people in homelike hospice residences, nursing homes, assisted living facilities, veterans' facilities, hospitals, and prisons.[1] Palliative care services are often provided initially as part of an acute care hospital stay and may be organized around an interdisciplinary consultation service with or without an acute inpatient palliative care ward. Palliative care may also be provided in the dying person's home as a "bridge" program between traditional home care services and hospice care, or it can be provided in long-term care facilities. In contrast, more than 80% of hospice care in the United States is provided in a patient's home, with the remainder provided to patients residing in long-term care facilities or in free-standing hospice residential facilities.[1] Hospice should be considered if the extent of disease and rate of decline indicate that the patient is likely to die within 6 months.

Why Is Palliative Care Appropriate for Neuromuscular Disease

Severely progressive neuromuscular disease (NMDs), including disorders like amyotrophic lateral sclerosis (ALS), spinal muscular atrophy, and Duchenne muscular dystrophy (DMD), pose unusual medical, ethical, and humanitarian considerations for the patient, the family, and the health care staff that are involved in their care.[3–9] These patients often have high symptom burdens, including chronic pain, muscle cramping, fatigue, dyspnea, and constipation, among others. Moreover, these patients and their families must make challenging decisions regarding the potential use of life-prolonging therapies, such as mechanical ventilation. The significant portion of the impact may be felt by family caregivers who are simultaneously struggling with arduous physical, emotional, and financial stressors associated with the NMD. Although these diseases are considered to be fatal, unlike most cancers or other incurable illnesses, patients with advanced NMD may live for many years before succumbing. Despite our current research developments and the most aggressive treatment available, patients with these diseases will inexorably continue to debilitate as the disease progresses. However, the lack of available curative treatments does not mean that physicians should take a nihilistic attitude, because palliative care is an appropriate treatment of NMDs. Optimal care should maximize function and quality of life for patients with an NMD. Expert multidisciplinary care may improve both quality and length of life of patients with progressive NMD.[10] Early involvement of palliative care specialists as part of the multidisciplinary team is theorized to likely improve the quality of life for patients with an NMD and their families, although this remains poorly studied.[11]

Depending on the subtype, an NMD may encompass many conditions, each with differing presentations, symptoms, and complexities. People with an advanced NMD often have insufficient care during the last year or so of life.[12–15] This infers that they may not have had a "good death" or did not die where they would have wished. People who are housebound cannot, by definition, attend clinic but they are seldom assessed at home either. Pain and other symptoms are often not adequately assessed or treated. Krivickas and colleagues[16] studied home care in 98 patients with ALS. In that sample, 24 were receiving nonhospice home care, 9 were receiving hospice home care, and 7 were receiving both hospice and nonhospice home care. Remarkably, 58 patients received no outside help. Patients receiving hospice were older than those receiving nonhospice home care (68.9 vs 57.7 years, $P<.05$). Patients with home care assistance had a mean ALS Functional Rating score of 13, and those without home care assistance had a mean score of 26 ($P<.0001$). Patients receiving nonhospice home care assistance received a median of 16 hours of care per week, whereas those with hospice received 5.5 hours of care per week ($P = .05$). Patients on Medicaid received more hours of home care than those with any other in-surance (median 61 vs 3.4 h/wk with Medicare and 5 h/wk with commercial insurance, $P = .008$). Not surprisingly, primary caregivers spent a median of 11 h/d caring for patients despite having home care assistance, and 42 (48%) of these primary care-givers felt physically ill and psychologically "burned out." This study clearly identified that home care received by patients with advanced ALS is inadequate and too late to relieve the burden placed on family caregivers.

A ROLE FOR PALLIATIVE CARE
How Palliative Care Can Help

Unlike hospice, palliative care is applicable early in the course of illness, in conjunction with other therapies that may indeed prolong life. The key to effective palliative care is communication. It is essential to ensure that the patient with NMD is able to under-stand as much as he or she wants to know about the disease and to be aware of what may happen as his or her disease progresses. This enables the patient to feel empowered to make informed choices regarding future care. This must be a 2-way process, with the person feeling that his or her views and preferences have been heard and understood by the clinician.

The basic tenets of palliative care include providing relief from pain, shortness of breath, nausea, and other distressing symptoms. This is done in the context of affirm-ing life yet acknowledging that dying is a normal process. The intent of palliative care is to neither hasten nor postpone death but instead to offer a support system to help patients live as fully as possible through the integration of medical, biopsychosocial, and spiritual aspects of patient care. This involves a multidisciplinary team to provide care for the patient. In this setting, pain is not simply treated as a singular entity but is approached as the sum of 4 components: physical noxious stimuli, affect or emotional discomfort, interpersonal conflicts, and the psychological aspects of accepting one's own death. These 4 components may individually or in combination affect patients' perception of their total pain. Failure on the physicians' part to fully understand and address each of these 4 components may result in less-than-optimal pain manage-ment at this stage of illness.

What Are the Challenges That Need to Be Addressed?

Given the advancements in health care, people with even severe NMDs like DMD are living longer now, often well in to adulthood, yet the need for care increases with time.[17–19] Young adults with DMD often report high life satisfaction.[20–23] Ideally, access and use of services increase in tandem with disease severity. However, this is not necessarily the case. Parker and colleagues[24] found discrepancies in service use in their study of 25 adult patients with DMD. Medical care and other services may lag behind increases in severity for a variety of reasons. For example, the family may not be aware of existing services or they may not understand the medical implications of a young patient's increased disease severity. Availability of services, distance to care, family resources, and transportation may all serve as barriers to care. Ideally, the need for services should predict their use; family resources, for example, should not factor into this. The need for services should equate roughly to disease severity, whereas limited family resources and lack of knowledge of available resources reflect inequitable access to these services. Yet service use models typically explain no more than 25% of the variance, whether predicting the use of individual services or the total number of services. Prior studies have shown considerable variance in other disabled patient populations in terms of use of palliative care services.[25–29] Family resources should not serve as barriers to palliative care services because insurance should cover most of these costs. The ability to access palliative care may be more dependent on patient and caregiver knowledge of what is available. Patients with NMD may not be aware of all services that are available that could potentially help them through the advanced stages of the disease process. Given that service use seems to be based more on resources and/or greater knowledge than on need is inequitable. Clearly, this dictates policy changes that include strategies to increase awareness of available services for all patients with NMD.

There are many other unanswered questions, including what aspects of care matter most for patients with an NMD who are receiving palliative services and what are the most effective strategies to alleviate suffering in patients with an NMD. Research has yet to identify the best practice standards in pain and symptom management for patients with an NMD with chronic pain who are in a palliative medicine program. The available literature indicates that patients with an advanced NMD have frequent, unplanned hospital admissions, which increase as the disease progresses.[30–32] Many factors account for this, including the long and unpredictable duration of advanced NMDs, the wide range of symptoms, the complex multidisciplinary care issues in DMD and ALS, neuropsychiatric problems (eg, behavioral and cognitive changes) that may negatively affect communication and care planning, and the common use of assisted ventilation aids in patients with NMD. It is worth considering that many patients with an NMD die of comorbid problems, instead of the disease itself. That is, they die with, but not of, their neuromuscular condition. This highlights the need, in the more rapidly advancing diseases, to obtain palliative care involved early in the disease progression.

How can end-of-life care be improved for people with an NMD? Communication is critical. Listen to what the person has to say about his or her own problems, strengths, and circumstances. The clinician must adequately assess the current problems and look for viable solutions. The multidisciplinary team should manage symptoms as part of holistic care. This improves an individual's quality of life and can ease burden on the family, both before and after death.[33,34]

Consider advance care planning, including advance decisions to refuse treatment and lasting power of attorney, and sensitively discuss with the person and caregivers their future care options. Clinicians can initiate open discussion around end-of-life care (ie, when talking about potentially life-prolonging treatment). However, the clinician must recognize that the person could die soon, thus justifying a more palliative approach. If a clinician is not used to thinking in these terms, he or she should ask himself or herself, "Considering the extent of disease, and rate of decline, would you be surprised if this person died in the next year?" If the answer is no, this would not be surprising and is expected; then consider introducing advance care planning and initiate discussions about managing the time the patient has left to them. For most clinicians, including most physicians, this involves a major paradigm shift in thinking. Physicians are often not very skilled at detecting subtle signs that would indicate that a palliative approach or even end-of-life care might be more appropriate and have not received training in how to approach these often very sensitive, uncomfortable discussions.

Possible triggers that indicate it is time to consider a palliative care approach for a patient with advanced NMD include (1) a marked decline in pulmonary function, particularly forced vital capacity and peak cough flow; (2) marked weight loss; (3) recurrent infections (typically pulmonary or urinary); (4) inability to heal lesions, including pressure ulcers; (5) swallowing problems; and (6) cognitive decline.

The savvy clinician will prepare the patient with an NMD well in advance of late-stage disease and facilitate end-of-life discussions by posing questions such as, "If you were to get a serious infection, where would you like to be treated?" "How aggressively do you want to be treated?" "Do you want all available medical interventions, including those that may be life prolonging?" Done properly, these questions would be asked when the patient is stable and doing well. The patient and family may need coaching, education, and time to consider the differing options and care pathways. Avoiding these conversations, whether early or late in the disease process, does the patient a disservice and may result in the loss of autonomy when, in the setting of an acute problem such as aspiration or sepsis, the person ends up being hospitalized and is given aggressive life-prolonging treatment, regardless of preference.

The Next Step: Integration of Palliative Care in NMD Management

We hope that we have presented a clear and logical argument that allows the reader to recognize need for palliative care in the management of progressive NMD. It is a better way to manage the complexity of care in this patient population. Although there is a great need for prospective research in this area, a recent study published in *The New England Journal of Medicine* showed that patients with lung cancer who received early palliative care experienced less depression and increased quality of life and survived almost 3 months longer than those receiving standard oncologic care.[35] We can do the same for palliative care in NMDs.

On the other hand, barriers still exist. Given the qualitative nature of these modalities of treatment, palliative care research has been hampered by methodologic challenges.[36–38] Much of this relates to variations in clinical trial design and care strategies, attrition, and missing data caused by patient death. The variation in palliative interventions and the wide variations in focus and extent of services make comparisons across trials difficult. Despite these limitations, accumulating evidence confirms that palliative care interventions improve patients' quality of life, satisfaction with care, and end-of-life outcomes.

Patients with incurable NMDs experience a considerable burden of physical and psychological distress, which often negatively impacts their quality of life. Palliative care clinicians are ideally suited to alleviate this suffering and to help patients with an NMD make informed decisions to direct their health care toward maximizing quality of life and improving satisfaction with care, family caregiver outcomes, health service use, and quality of end-of-life care.

REFERENCES

1. Smith TJ, Temin S, Alesi ER, et al. American Society of Clinical Oncology provisional clinical opinion: the integration of palliative care into standard oncology care. J Clin Oncol 2012;30(8):880–7.

2. Zimmermann C, Riechelmann R, Krzyzanowska M, et al. Effectiveness of specialized palliative care: a systematic review. JAMA 2008;299(14):1698–709.

3. McDonald CM, Abresch RT, Carter GT, et al. Profiles of neuromuscular disease: Duchenne muscular dystrophy. Am J Phys Med Rehabil 1995;74(5):S70–92.

4. McDonald CM, Abresch RT, Carter GT, et al. Profiles of neuromuscular disease: Becker muscular dystrophy. Am J Phys Med Rehabil 1995;74(5):S93–103.

5. Johnson ER, Carter GT, Kilmer DD, et al. Profiles of neuromuscular disease: myotonic muscular dystrophy. Am J Phys Med Rehabil 1995;74(5):S104–16.

6. McDonald CM, Abresch RT, Carter GT, et al. Profiles of neuromuscular disease: limb-girdle syndromes. Am J Phys Med Rehabil 1995;74(5):S117–30.

7. Kilmer DD, Abresch RT, Aitkens SG, et al. Profiles of neuromuscular disease: facioscapulohumeral dystrophy. Am J Phys Med Rehabil 1995;74(5):S131–9.

8. Carter GT, Abresch RT, Fowler WM, et al. Profiles of neuromuscular disease: hereditary motor and sensory neuropathy, types I and II. Am J Phys Med Rehabil 1995;74(5):S140–9.

9. Carter GT, Abresch RT, Fowler WM, et al. Profiles of neuromuscular disease: spinal muscular atrophy. Am J Phys Med Rehabil 1995;74(5):S150–9.

10. Fowler WM, Carter GT, Kraft GH. Role of physiatry in the management of neuromuscular disease. Phys Med Rehabil Clin N Am 1998;9(1):1–8.

11. Mayadev AS, Weiss MD, Distad BJ, et al. The amyotrophic lateral sclerosis center: a model of multidisciplinary management. Phys Med Rehabil Clin N Am 2008;19(3):619–31.

12. Carter GT, Butler LM, Abresch RT, et al. Expanding the role of hospice in the care of amyotrophic lateral sclerosis. Am J Hosp Palliat Care 1999;16(6):707–10.

13. Bernat JL. Ethical and legal issues in the management of amyotrophic lateral sclerosis. In: Belsh JM, Schiffman PL, editors. Amyotrophic lateral sclerosis: diagnosis and management for the clinician. Armonk (NY): Futura; 1996. p. 357–72.

14. Ganzini L, Johnston WS, McFarland BH, et al. Attitudes of patients with amyotrophic lateral sclerosis and their caregivers toward assisted suicide. N Engl J Med 1998;339(14):967–73.

15. Moore MK. Dying at home: a way of maintaining control for the person with ALS/MND. Palliat Med 1993;7(Suppl 4):65–8.

16. Krivickas LS, Shockley L, Mitsumoto H. Homecare of patients with amyotrophic lateral sclerosis (ALS). J Neurol Sci 1997;152(Suppl 1(2)):S82–9.

17. Eagle M, Baudouin SV, Chandler C, et al. Survival in Duchenne muscular dystrophy: improvements in life expectancy since 1967 and the impact of home nocturnal ventilation. Neuromuscul Disord 2002;12(10):926–9.

18. Kohler M, Clarenback CF, Bahler C, et al. Disability and survival in Duchenne muscular dystrophy. J Neurol Neurosurg Psychiatr 2009;80(3):320–5.

19. Fraser LK, Childs AM, Miller M, et al. A cohort study of children and young people with progressive neuromuscular disorders: clinical and demographic profiles and changing patterns of referral for palliative care. Palliat Med 2011. [Epub ahead of print].

20. Miller JR, Colbert AP, Osberg JS. Ventilator dependency: decision-making, daily functioning and quality of life for patients with Duchenne muscular dystrophy. Dev Med Child Neurol 1990;32(12):1078–86.

21. Bach JR, Campagnolo DI, Hoeman S. Life satisfaction of individuals with Duchenne muscular dystrophy using long-term mechanical ventilatory support. Am J Phys Med Rehabil 1991;70(3):129–35.

22. Kohler M, Clarenback CF, Boni L, et al. Quality of life, physical disability, and respiratory impairment in Duchenne muscular dystrophy. Am J Respir Crit Care Med 2005;172(8):1032–6.

23. Carter GT, Weiss MD, Chamberlain JR, et al. Aging in muscular dystrophy: pathophysiology and clinical management. Phys Med Rehabil Clin N Am 2010;21(2): 429–50.

24. Parker AE, Robb SA, Chambers J, et al. Analysis of an adult Duchenne muscular dystrophy population. QJM 2005;98(10):729–36.

25. Bass DM, Noelker LS. The influence of family caregivers on elders' use of inhome services: an expanded conceptual framework. J Health Soc Behav 1987;28(2): 184–96.

26. Balkrishnan R, Naughton M, Smith BP, et al. Parent caregiver-related predictors of health care service utilization by children with cerebral palsy enrolled in Medicaid. J Pediatr Health Care 2002;16(2):73–8.

27. Smith GC. Aging families of adults with mental retardation: patterns and correlates of service use, need, and knowledge. Am J Ment Retard 1997;102(1):13–26.

28. Maganã S, Seltzer MM, Krauss MW. Service utilization patterns of adults with intellectual disabilities: a comparison of Puerto Rican and non-Latino white families. J Gerontol Soc Work 2002;37(3–4):65–86.

29. Pruchno RA, McMullen WF. Patterns of service utilization by adults with a developmental disability: type of service makes a difference. Am J Ment Retard 2004; 109(5):362–78.

30. Arias R, Andrews J, Pandya S, et al. Palliative care services in families of males with Duchenne muscular dystrophy. Muscle Nerve 2011;44(1):93–101.

31. Bede P, Oliver D, Stodart J, et al. Palliative care in amyotrophic lateral sclerosis: a review of current international guidelines and initiatives. J Neurol Neurosurg Psychiatry 2011;82(4):413–8.

32. Blackhall LJ. Amyotrophic lateral sclerosis and palliative care: where we are, and the road ahead. Muscle Nerve 2012;45(3):311–8.

33. Baumrucker SJ, Stolick M, Carter GT, et al. Death, dying, and statistics: quality measures versus quality of life. Am J Hosp Palliat Med 2010;27(7):494–9.

34. Enck RE. Hospice: the next step. Am J Hosp Palliat Care 1999;16(2):436–7.

35. Temel JS, Greer JA, Muzikansky A, et al. Early palliative care for patients with metastatic non–small-cell lung cancer. N Engl J Med 2010;363:733–42.

36. Greer JA, Pirl WF, Jackson VA, et al. Effect of early palliative care on chemotherapy use and end-of-life care in patients with metastatic non-small-cell lung cancer. J Clin Oncol 2012;30(4):394–400.

37. El-Jawahri A, Greer JA, Temel JS. Does palliative care improve outcomes for patients with incurable illness? A review of the evidence. J Support Oncol 2011;9(3):87–94.

38. von Gunten CF. Evolution and effectiveness of palliative care. Am J Geriatr Psychiatry 2012;20(4):291–7.

Index

Note: Page numbers of article titles are in **boldface** type.

Phys Med Rehabil Clin N Am 23 (2012) 911–922
http://dx.doi.org/10.1016/S1047-9651(12)00109-X
1047-9651/12/$ – see front matter © 2012 Elsevier Inc. All rights reserved.